"Less than a chapter in, I already knew I'd be recommending this book to ᵃ
read a LOT of acceptance and commitment therapy (ACT) workbooks in my
practitioner, and this is one of the very best. A must-have for anyone lookinᵍ
chological flexibility skills for a well-lived life."

    —**Jill Stoddard, PhD**, coauthor of *The Big Book of ACT Metaphors*

"*The Acceptance and Commitment Therapy Skills Workbook* is a superb guide to building a better life. With
a compassionate, wise, and easy-to-understand writing style, the authors introduce you to a wide range of
powerful tools and strategies that can help just about anyone to reduce suffering and make life richer and
fuller. Highly recommended!"

    —**Russ Harris,** author of *The Happiness Trap* and *ACT Made Simple*

"This is an excellent resource for the many professionals who work in primary care and general practice
clinics. So many people come to their doctors with emotional pain, and this book can help them and their
behavioral health teammates recognize and address that pain. So, if you have emotional pain, read this
book and tell your doctor! Thanks, Matt and Jen, for a concise and powerful book that can alleviate suffering at many levels."

    —**Patricia Robinson, PhD**, president of Mountainview Consulting Group,
      and author of *Behavioral Consultation and Primary Care*

"If you were going to buy just one book to help you flourish both on the inside and the outside, *The
Acceptance and Commitment Therapy Skills Workbook* would be it! Beautifully written in a humble, straight-
forward way, this book is chock-full of practical ideas and personal growth exercises that will carry you
through life's ups and downs. Take this gift home with you and unwrap it into your life!"

    —**Kirk D. Strosahl, PhD**, coauthor of *The Mindfulness and Acceptance Workbook for Depression*

"'*It's kinda lovely here.*' Join the authors as they help you embrace your humanity, face struggles, and live
according to what matters to you. This book gives you the best evidence-based strategies to travel along
the valued life journey. It's practical and written by folks who are the real deal. They've helped thousands
of people and found their way through their own struggles to a life lived well."

    —**Louise L. Hayes, PhD,** coauthor of *What Makes You Stronger* and *Your Life Your, Way*;
      developer of DNA-V; and clinical psychologist and adjunct senior research fellow
      at La Trobe University, Melbourne

"Boone and Gregg have created a really accessible, transdiagnostic self-help workbook grounded in ACT. It offers practical guidance to address a range of emotional struggles, helping you cultivate mindfulness, embrace your values, and navigate life's challenges with greater resilience. With a gentle and compassionate approach, this book serves as a beacon for those seeking a more meaningful and authentic life."

—**Kelly G. Wilson, PhD**, professor emeritus at the University of Mississippi,
and coauthor of *Mindfulness for Two* and *Acceptance and Commitment Therapy*

"An extremely friendly and approachable introduction to the core concepts of ACT. The authors have done a spectacular job of taking complex material and making it accessible, useful, and fun. I learned a lot and will take these exercises and ideas into my daily life. I especially enjoyed the chapter on gratitude, awe, and savoring. What a wonderful addition to the ACT literature! Read this book. You'll get a lot out of it."

—**Spencer Smith**, coauthor of *Get Out of Your Mind and Into Your Life*

"In this excellent, very human, easily accessible, and deeply engaging book written by clinicians for all of us who struggle with feeling and thinking things we'd rather not, you will find the best of ACT distilled into clear, immediately usable, effective tools. Boone and Gregg have written a beautiful book that will be a fixture on your night table, or pulled off your shelf again and again. If I could put a book on speed dial, this would be it!"

—**Lisa W. Coyne, PhD**, assistant professor at Harvard Medical School,
and CEO of the New England Center for OCD and Anxiety

"*The Acceptance and Commitment Therapy Skills Workbook* is an insightful book offering a comprehensive approach to personal growth and emotional well-being. From mastering defusion and present-moment awareness to embracing willingness and aligning actions with values, each chapter is a stepping stone toward meaningful living. Matthew Boone and Jennifer Gregg have created an integrated process exploring perspective taking and positive psychology principles, empowering readers to cultivate resilience that supports living with greater flexibility and purpose. An essential read for anyone seeking transformation through ACT."

—**Robyn D. Walser, PhD**, licensed clinical psychologist, author of *The Heart of ACT*,
and coauthor of *Learning ACT*, *The Mindful Couple*, *Acceptance and Commitment Therapy for the Treatment of Post-Traumatic Stress Disorder and Trauma-Based Problems*,
and *The ACT Workbook for Anger*

The
Acceptance
& Commitment
Therapy Skills
WORKBOOK

Cope with Emotional Pain,
Connect with What Matters &
Transform Your Life

Matthew S. Boone, LCSW | Jennifer Gregg, PhD

New Harbinger Publications, Inc.

Publisher's Note

NEW HARBINGER PUBLICATIONS is a registered trademark of New Harbinger Publications, Inc.

New Harbinger Publications is an employee-owned company.

Copyright © 2024 by Matthew S. Boone and Jennifer Gregg

New Harbinger Publications, Inc.
5720 Shattuck Avenue
Oakland, CA 94609
www.newharbinger.com

Cover design by Amy Shoup

Acquired by Elizabeth Hollis Hansen

Edited by M. C. Calvi

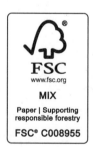

Printed in the United States of America

26   25   24

10   9   8   7   6   5   4   3   2   1   First Printing

For Jeptha T. Boone, MD (1935–2020), my father and my first and best model for caring for patients, serving my community, and being someone to go to when things are hard.

—MSB

For Glenn, my Steens, without whom this life would be nowhere near as amazing.

—JAG

Contents

Foreword

In today's world, most people know that mental resilience is a skill that needs to be cultivated. We may have learned to categorize mental struggles in the language of "illness" and "disorder," but the limits of that language are obvious when nearly everybody needs help to learn how to interact with the modern world in a way that creates more of a sense of peace, meaning, and connection.

As a result of this human need, there is an ever-expanding universe of psychotherapy and personal growth, with a cacophony of voices, theories, techniques, and manuals aplenty. Each claims to help users chart a course toward inner peace, self-acceptance, and a fulfilling life, but the strength of the evidence is often thin, and the reader has to trust that the processes being taught are truly central.

Every person who seeks out self-help has a right to expect that the methods being taught have been repeatedly shown to be helpful and that we know why these methods work. It sounds like a simple standard, but many of the approaches that are being popularized cannot meet them.

Acceptance and commitment therapy (or "ACT," said as a single word) more certainly can do so. There are over two hundred randomized controlled trials in top-ranked journals. The World Health Organization distributes ACT self-help based on extensive and successful empirical testing, and most of the major scientific organizations that determine if a method is evidence-based include ACT as one of their evidence-based methods. And there is arguably more and more supportive evidence of why ACT works than almost any other psychotherapy method.

ACT works by increasing psychological flexibility and by decreasing psychological inflexibility. What that means can be summarized in a simple sentence. The ACT literature shows that in order to prosper, we need to learn to be more emotionally and cognitively open, more consciously centered in the present moment, and more actively engaged in a values-based life.

The Acceptance and Commitment Therapy Skills Workbook teaches these skills. It traverses the human landscape of human emotion and cognition with a deftness and clarity born of lengthy clinical experience. The book is crafted by two world renowned ACT trainers: Jennifer Gregg, a clinical psychologist and my former student, and Matt Boone, a leading clinical social worker. They are known for their creativity, good humor, clinical skill, and compassion. All of these qualities are obvious and evident in the book itself.

Over four decades ago, when the seeds of ACT were first sown, they contained the promise of a more meaningful life and an embrace of all that it is to be human. Jennifer and Matthew, through this workbook, have cultivated those seeds. This is not a dry "thinkbook," nor a compendium of case studies. Neither is it the kind of rousing self-focused motivational rant that too often characterizes the self-help shelves. Instead, what unfolds within these pages is a creative, step-by-step journey toward acquiring the skills necessary for a more psychologically flexible life.

ACT is fundamentally experiential. Its potency lies not in a purely intellectual grasp of its principles, but in the lived and felt experience of their relevance to our lives. Jennifer and Matthew have harnessed this truth, presenting a multitude of active exercises arranged in a coherent step-by-step progression. The book is a call to self-exploration. The exercises are like steppingstones through a muddy field—a solid path to a life that is more heartfelt, more present, and more meaningful.

In my years of developing ACT, I have witnessed firsthand its profound impact on both clients and practitioners. This workbook encapsulates that impact in its essence. It breaks down the complexity of psychological flexibility into accessible "bite-size" chunks. The clinical expertise of the authors shines through not just in the substance of the exercises but in their delivery—infused with humor, compassion, and an undercurrent of support that makes the journey through these pages feel less like a solitary trek and more like a shared exploration.

One of the many strengths of this workbook is its refusal to succumb to a narrative voice that rises above the head of reader for fear of being seen. It does not posture as the all-knowing guide, from a lofty perch. Rather, it invites you to engage in a kind of heartfelt dialogue with the authors, a warm and witty conversation with wise companions who understand the terrain because they have walked this way before with others and—even more importantly—they are walking it beside you now.

An innovative aspect of the workbook is its embrace of positive psychology. In one of the last chapters, it urges the reader to expect more and to grow in positive directions—to savor life, to engender gratitude, and sit inside appreciation of life itself. That approach to psychological flexibility readily extends it into every corner of our lives and rounds out your work in learning how to be more flexible in an important way.

The Acceptance and Commitment Therapy Skills Workbook is, at its heart, an invitation—to self-discovery, self-kindness, and to a values-based life focused on others. As you turn the pages of this book, I encourage you to adopt a humble posture of curiosity, and to reignite the spark of wonder that you once had when you examined your world with eager eyes. Yes, you may be in pain—but that is a precious opportunity to learn anew how to be whole and free.

Let this workbook be a guide, a map, and a companion. If you sense deeply that it is time for you to take steps toward the values-based life you seek—one exercise, one moment, one breath at a time—you are in wonderful hands. I know it because I know these authors for the kind and extraordinarily capable professionals they are. You will soon know as well because you will sense what they are up to as human beings.

If you sense that now is the time for real change and for a new direction you have come to the right place. Your sense is correct. You landed here for a reason: It's time to begin.

—Steven C. Hayes, PhD

Foundation Professor of Psychology Emeritus

University of Nevada, Reno

President, Institute for Better Health

Originator of acceptance and commitment therapy

CHAPTER 1

Introducing Acceptance and Commitment Therapy

Being human is hard. No matter what we do, we'll all encounter our share of suffering. Though life will be joyous at times, it will also be painful. We'll experience losses, conflicts, illnesses, and life disruptions, and we won't be able to escape the inevitable pain that arises: sadness, anxiety, fear, shame, guilt, worries, difficult memories, thoughts that we are "not good enough," and on and on.

Yet, our conversations about hard things and the difficult feelings that accompany them—whether those conversations are with others or in our own heads—typically involve minimizing, ignoring, or overcoming them. "You just have to move on," "You're taking things too personally," "This will be good for you," "God never gives you anything you can't handle," "Suck it up and quit complaining," "Look on the bright side!" ad infinitum. Have you noticed that these ways of coping rarely help? Or if they motivate you a little bit, they also make you feel defective, like you shouldn't take it so hard?

If you're reading this book, you're either (1) looking for an alternative or (2) hoping to find a better way to push through. Either way, you're in the right place. We'd like to introduce (or reintroduce) you to acceptance and commitment therapy (ACT). ACT is a science-based model of behavior change and personal growth that starts from the assumption that life can be hard, and that difficult thoughts and feelings will inevitably arise. ACT offers a new perspective and useful skills for encountering life differently and making space for what's beautiful, amazing, and precious along the way.

Control Is the Problem, Not the Solution

ACT (said like the word "act," not three letters) has a lot of moving parts, but you really only need to know one thing before we dive in. ACT draws on a piece of wisdom about thoughts and feelings that most of us know but that we often forget:

If I asked you not to think of a white bear for the next thirty seconds, what do you think would happen?

Almost everyone gets this right. They usually smile knowingly and say something like, "I would think about white bears!" We all know this intuitively, and there's lots of science to support it (e.g., Wegner 1994; Wenzlaff and Wegner 2000). Yet, the very first thing we do when something uncomfortable shows up inside of us—shame, a negative thought, or some version of "I'm not good enough"—is to try to push it away.

This is called "thought suppression," and it's something we all do from time to time. Though it works sometimes, it doesn't work all the time. When it does work, that uncomfortable thought or feeling sometimes comes back—much stronger, even. And when thought suppression becomes one of our primary ways to deal with difficult thoughts and feelings, it can create bigger problems. Just think of the last time you put something important off by pushing it out of your mind. Did that make the problem go away?

Suppression is just one way that we try to exert control over our thoughts and feelings—to change them in some way when we don't want to deal with the discomfort they can cause us. There are lots of others: procrastinating, scrolling social media, giving ourselves pep talks, criticizing ourselves, imagining ways to escape, venting our feelings, worrying, bossing around friends and family, and on and on and on. These strategies are so automatic and so common that we rarely even notice that they are about trying to control—suppress, avoid, push away, or ignore—uncomfortable thoughts and feelings.

All these strategies work—to a point. All of them help us manage the difficulties that come our way—both in our lives and inside of ourselves. They're not wrong, and using them doesn't mean we're defective. But they can have real side effects. Here are a couple of examples—though they are not real people, they are very much like the people we talk to in our offices every day.

Camille feels anxious in groups, especially at work. She rarely goes out with her colleagues and doesn't speak up in meetings. She doesn't want people to see her face flushing when she talks, and she doesn't like the feeling of her heart racing. As a result, she feels disconnected from her colleagues, who don't really know her—or her great ideas—very well. And the anxiety persists.

Feliciano feels embarrassed when he misses a shot or makes a bad pass during pickup basketball. So, he criticizes himself for his mistakes and chastises himself for feeling embarrassed, seeing both as weak. This motivates him, but it also makes him feel guilty for feeling embarrassed, and he loses focus, leading to further mistakes and, unsurprisingly, more embarrassment.

Tanya never feels good enough in her college classes and constantly compares herself to her peers. So, she studies constantly, never taking breaks, and never taking advantage of all the extracurricular experiences college has to offer. She gets good grades, but she's always exhausted and sleep deprived, has a nagging sense that she is missing out on things, and never seems to shake the "not good enough" feeling.

See the pattern? Camille, Feliciano, and Tanya all feel bad about something. They do something to try not to feel bad. It works a little, but things ultimately stay the same or even get worse. This pattern of human behavior is so common that it's got a name: *experiential avoidance*. They are trying to avoid or control uncomfortable internal experiences—anxiety and its attendant physical sensations, embarrassment, or the thought of "not good enough"—and doing so leads to further problems. This is something everyone does to some degree. But we often don't notice it in our own lives. Check in with yourself: do these patterns sound familiar to you?

Let's not just talk about it. This is a workbook, after all, so before we go much further, let's *do* a little bit of ACT. ACT is an experiential approach, which means its lessons are best learned by experiencing them, not just talking or reading about them.

EXERCISE: How Well Does Control Work for You?

In the left column of the following chart, write a list of all the thoughts and feelings you'd like to get rid of. Make sure to include stuff your mind says and does (e.g., "not good enough," worrying, rehashing past hurts), emotions (e.g., anxiety, shame, sadness), and body sensations (e.g., racing heart, feeling shaky, upset stomach). See if you can avoid writing down difficult *situations*, such as an annoying family member. Instead, write your reactions to those situations, such as irritability.

Then, in the right column, write a list of all the things you do or have done in the past to try to make those thoughts and feelings go away. Make sure to include both the things you might be proud of (e.g., going to therapy) and those that you're not (e.g., procrastinating, doomscrolling social media). Also, make sure to include things you've done mentally, such as criticizing yourself, problem solving, and worrying.

Here's a list of the types of things that people tend put in this chart, if you need examples:

Thoughts and feelings I'd like to get rid of		Things I've done to try to make them go away	
Stress	Butterflies	Exercise	Go to the gym
Worry	Heaviness	Eating too much or too little	Porn
Overwhelm	"Not good enough"		Read
Burnout	"Not fair"	Procrastination	Self-help books
Shame	"Never get it right"	Worry	Self-help apps
Boredom	"People are bad"	Problem solving	Therapy
Anger	"Stuck in a rut"	Criticize myself	Medication
Helplessness	"It's not right!" "If only…"	Criticize others	Sleep
Hopelessness		Drink alcohol	Cannabis
Exhaustion	"Should do better"	Isolate	CBD
Busy mind	Painful memories	Pray	Talk to friends
Revved up	Impostor thoughts	Meditate	Journal
Anxiety	Urge to drink	Yoga	Avoid
Lack of motivation	Physical pain	Netflix	Procrastinate
Back pain	Pit in my stomach	Social media	Watch TV
Upset stomach	Lump in my throat	Plan	Practice gratitude
		Take deep breaths	

Thoughts and feelings I'd like to get rid of	Things I've done to try to make them go away

Once you have some items written down, underline everything in the right column that works in the short term to make the stuff in the left column go away. "The short term" means any time from right away to within a few hours.

Next, circle everything in the right column that works in the long term to make the stuff in the left column go away. "The long term" means they go away and never come back.

Reflection: What do you notice about the difference between the strategies that help in the short term and in the long term?

_____

_____

_____

_____

_____

_____

_____

You probably noticed that just about everything on the right side makes a difference in the short term. And if it doesn't now, it might have in the past. That makes sense: we typically don't do things that don't have some kind of impact. What we do works for us, or we wouldn't do it. (Obviously, it's more complicated than that, and we will touch on that complexity later.)

You probably also noticed that none of those strategies really make anything on the left go away in the long term—since we're defining that to mean "goes away and never comes back." It's also possible you circled things like "meditate" and "therapy." Though those activities can help you build a richer, more meaningful life, they can't really keep painful thoughts and feelings from showing up either, though we often assume they will.

Shifting Perspective

Let's add one final part to this exercise, one that shifts our perspective a bit: Put a star by everything in the right column that brings you closer to a rich, meaningful, well-lived life. Don't think too hard about what that means just yet, just go with your gut. When you're done, come back to the question below.

Reflection: What do you notice about the things you starred?

_____

_____

_____

_____

_____

_____

_____

_____

Below are some things you might have noticed, as well as some points we'd invite you to consider if you haven't already.

1. It's likely that far fewer of the things on the right are starred than are underlined. If you're like most people, your behavior can easily fall into persistent patterns of trying to feel okay at the expense of things you care about.

2. There might be some other things you would add to the list of actions that help you build a meaningful life. Remember those for later!

3. Almost anything on the right can bring you closer to a rich, meaningful, well-lived life—depending on the circumstances. Let's take "talking to friends," for example. Imagine a scenario in which venting to a friend helps you feel seen and heard, offers your friend an opportunity to support you, and strengthens your connection. Then, imagine one in which venting just makes you more frustrated, leaves your friend exhausted, and creates separation between you. Both are potential outcomes of the same action—venting—under different circumstances.

Another example might be drinking alcohol. Imagine a scenario in which having a few drinks is about celebrating the end of a big project or enhancing a delicious meal. Then, imagine one in which having a couple of drinks is part of a persistent, anxiety-driven pattern of trying to avoid problems and quiet a worried mind.

The point is that, from an ACT perspective, behaviors themselves are neither bad nor good, healthy nor unhealthy. It all depends on context: what's the situation? Who is the person behaving? What's the history of that behavior in their life? How does it impact them and the people around them?

ACT invites you to sharpen your awareness of how your actions operate. You might ask: is this behavior, in this moment, about avoiding or controlling uncomfortable thoughts and feelings? Is it about building a rich, meaningful, well-lived life? Or a little of both? If you can ask these questions—first very explicitly, then over time more implicitly—you can start making changes.

As you ask these questions, it's also helpful to consider not just how your behavior works, but also what it might be costing you in your life: your career, your relationships, your ability to enjoy yourself, or the way you feel from day to day.

The Cost of Control

Take another look at the previous exercise again—specifically, look at the list in the righthand column. Let's call these "control strategies." Pick out four to five control strategies you use that you suspect are not serving you well. In the space below, elaborate on what they cost you in your life—in other words, the impact they have over the long term that might be making things worse for you.

If you'd like examples, you can see some from Camille, Feliciano, and Tanya, the folks we described a little bit earlier, after the next table.

EXERCISE: The Cost of Control

Control strategy Stuff I do to avoid and control uncomfortable thoughts and feelings	Cost The impact these control strategies have over the long term

Camille's Costs of Control

Control strategy	Cost
Stuff I do to avoid and control uncomfortable thoughts and feelings	The impact these control strategies have over the long term
I rarely go out with work colleagues.	They don't really invite me anymore. It seems like they're having fun and I'm missing out. I don't feel like I know them very well.
I rarely speak up in meetings.	I continue to be uncomfortable in meetings because I don't have any practice speaking my mind. Also, my colleagues might think I don't contribute much.

Feliciano's Costs of Control

Control strategy	Cost
Stuff I do to avoid and control uncomfortable thoughts and feelings	The impact these control strategies have over the long term
When I make a mistake and feel embarrassed, I criticize myself for being weak.	I feel worse, and I'm always in my head when I'm on the court. I think it affects how I perform, and I don't really enjoy myself unless I never make a mistake.

Tanya's Costs of Control

Control strategy	Cost
Stuff I do to avoid and control uncomfortable thoughts and feelings	The impact these control strategies have over the long term
I work all the time to try not to feel so anxious.	I feel anxious anyway, and I'm never really pleased with my successes. Also, I'm missing out on a lot of parts of college: friends, new experiences, fun.

Don't worry if you don't think you've identified all the costs. This is just a rough draft, so to speak. The practice of ACT involves learning to open your eyes to the way control plays out in your life. You will learn more and more as you go.

Letting Go of Control

Before we go any further, let's debrief a little bit. What are you noticing about the ACT perspective on how control plays out in people's lives?

_____

_____

_____

_____

_____

_____

_____

_____

Folks we work with have a variety of reactions to these first couple of exercises, just like you might have. There's no right response, but we'd like to speak to a few you might be having.

Guilt or shame. Some people feel guilt or shame, as if they've done something wrong by falling into these patterns of avoidance and control. We are here to tell you that there's nothing wrong with you. This is a very human way to respond. Most of us fall into some version of this pattern almost every day. You're in good company.

Sadness. Many people feel some sadness as they notice this pattern. They identify meaningful things that they have given up on or let go of in the interest of trying to feel "okay." Sadness is a very important emotion—it tells us what we care about. If you're feeling sadness, we feel for you. Do your best to treat this sadness as good information, and don't let it spiral into self-criticism or hopelessness for the future. This book may be able to help you make your future different.

Relief. Some people feel relief. They realize that they are not failures—they are *not* the only people who struggle with these thoughts and feelings, and they are not the only people who give over some part of their life to this struggle. If you're feeling relief, we're glad. Welcome to the human condition!

A sense of commonality with other people. Yes! We all do this sort of thing. It's hard to connect to this sense of commonality when you do an exercise like this by yourself, but when we do this exercise in groups, people often feel less alone, more connected to the people around them. They think to themselves, "I'm not the only one who does this! We all hurt, and we all fall into patterns of unnecessarily trying to control our thoughts and feelings." In fact, the examples we offered you in the first exercise come from the therapy clients we work with, the mental health professionals we train, and our own lives.

If we haven't anticipated any of your responses, that's okay. Whatever you feel is normal. We are not just saying that. Really, you are entitled to your reactions, no matter what they are. This book is about learning how to respond differently to your reactions so that they don't have an unnecessary impact on your life.

Workability

By the way, letting go of control doesn't mean completely banishing efforts to avoid or control uncomfortable thoughts and feelings altogether. That would be impossible—this pattern of behavior is so ingrained, it's likely to stick around throughout your life. Also, as we noted, some behaviors sort of work, don't have meaningful negative consequences, and can even be about building a life of meaning and vitality. So, the goal of ACT is not to give up all control strategies. Instead, what we'd like you to learn to do over the course of this book is become more aware of how your behavior works, so that you can make a conscious choice when you act.

So, for example, you might pick up a drink and ask, "What is this about for me right now?" And with that knowledge, you can choose to take that drink or not, depending on how it works for you and your life.

Or you might be tempted to vent to a friend, but first ask yourself, "What is this about for me right now?" and, with that knowledge, make a conscious choice.

In ACT, we call this *workability*. ACT invites you to assess how a behavior works for you in at least two domains: what you're going after in this moment *and* the big picture of building a rich, meaningful, well-lived life.

Okay, let's get back to control.

Why Do We Work So Hard to Control?

These automatic and often unconscious efforts to control thoughts and feelings are thought to be the result of evolution. Early humans on the African savanna used feelings as information. If they felt scared, that meant there was likely danger, and they had to do something about it by running, fighting, or hiding. If they felt hunger, they had to do something about it by finding something to eat. And if they felt ashamed or guilty for going against the customs of the small groups they lived in and counted on for survival, they needed to take action to rebuild their relationships. Their emotions told them they needed to do something, and if they didn't try to do it, they might not survive.

In contemporary life, most of us are not at risk of starvation, bodily harm, or rejection from our social groups on a daily basis. Sadly, that's not true for everybody, but it's a reality for many of us. But even when we're relatively safe and sound, our thoughts and feelings are still built to keep us alive in the face of daily threats, and our action tendencies often serve their demands. So, if we feel anxious, then we need to do something to make the anxiety dissipate. If we feel sad, we need to do something to attend to that sadness. And if we feel ashamed, we need to do something to attenuate that shame. It's just that automatic, even if it doesn't always work for our lives.

It's also true that just because we're not facing the direct threats early humans might have faced, that doesn't mean adversity or suffering aren't part of our lives. It turns out that going through hard stuff is just part of the human condition. So, if you're reading this book because you're struggling in some way, and you've been told or you feel that ACT will help, you're in good company.

Suffering Is Part of the Human Condition

Every year, one in five people will qualify for a diagnosis of a mental health problem like depression, anxiety, or substance use disorder. One in five! Over the course of our lives, 46 percent of us—nearly half—will deal with one of these problems (McGrath et al. 2023). And these data don't take into account the variety of ways that we can feel overwhelmed that don't necessarily lead to a diagnosis—breakups, births, deaths, natural disasters, bad jobs, new jobs, family conflict, and on and on.

You could look at these data and think, "Dang, there's an epidemic of mental health problems in the world!" And you'd be in good company—there's research supporting the concern that these numbers are going up, especially since the beginning of the pandemic (WHO 2022). But you could also look at these data and come to a different conclusion: being human is hard and hurting is part of the human condition, and these data represent the natural variation of human experience. We will all feel anxious. We will all feel depressed. We will all struggle with something, perhaps many times across the course of our lives.

This isn't the end of the story, however. This book isn't about resigning yourself to difficulty and just toughing it out. As the name "acceptance and commitment therapy" would imply, it's about understanding this part of reality, deciding what you'll *do* once you've acknowledged it, and committing to brave action in service of what you most value in life. And ACT offers you a bunch of ways to navigate the hard stuff when it arises, as it inevitably will. One of the most important ways is to tie the hard stuff to what you care about in life, a skill which we will briefly introduce you to next.

Values: The Way We Live Well

ACT invites you to identify your values—what you really care about in life—and then consciously choose actions that serve those values, no matter what thoughts and feelings show up along the way. In a sense, instead of helping you "feel good," ACT encourages you to live well. So instead of asking yourself, "How can I get rid of this anxiety?" you might ask, "What would I be doing right now if anxiety wasn't in charge? What would I be doing right now if I was focusing on what matters to me?"

The focus on values over controlling thoughts and feelings doesn't mean that ACT teaches you to just suck it up and push through. "Acceptance" in ACT doesn't mean giving up, giving in, or resigning yourself to a bad situation. And it doesn't mean gritting your teeth in a "no pain, no gain" kind of way.

Instead, ACT invites us to acknowledge that if we are going to live a meaningful life—be part of a community, pursue a meaningful career, build a family, look for fun and adventure, or whatever else we care about—then life will be both beautiful and hard. And values offer us a framework for navigating the hard stuff. Check in with yourself: when something is difficult, might it be easier to do if it's connected to something meaningful to you? Isn't it just a little bit easier to study for that exam if it's about building a career that you want, rather than because you *have to*? Isn't it just a little bit easier to get up in the morning and take your kids to school because you want to be the best parent you can be?

ACT brings this perspective to handling thoughts and feelings: what if all the stuff you'd rather not have inside you—anxiety, sadness, self-critical thoughts, difficulty trusting other people, or fear that you'll never measure up—could be carried in the service of what you care about most deeply in life? Might that be worth it? If you continue through this book, you might just discover that it is.

By the way, the emphasis on living well over feeling good doesn't mean that people who adopt ACT as a way of coping—whether in therapy, coaching, an app, or a self-help book—don't feel better. For the most part, they do. In studies, ACT tends to do just as well at reducing depression, anxiety, stress, and whatever else people struggle with as other well-researched therapies (Gloster et al. 2020). It's just that in ACT, feeling better is a byproduct of showing up to thoughts and feelings with mindfulness and kindness while focusing on living well. But let's be honest: no one would do it if they didn't get some relief.

Experiencing relief from what you suffer with is a gift, and we don't mean to downplay it. Anyone who is suffering wants relief. But if that's all life has to offer, then that might be a pretty dull life. Life is about more than feeling good or feeling bad. Life is about living.

Psychological Flexibility

Living meaningfully while carrying your pain with kindness is called "psychological flexibility." Over the course of the next eight chapters, we will introduce you to different ways to become more flexible, based on the different components of psychological flexibility that are taught in ACT. And in each chapter, you'll find a bunch of exercises, techniques, and practices to help you bring each component to life. Let's take a moment and go over these different components right now.

Defusion. Defusion involves becoming intimately acquainted with what your mind does without getting swept away in it. So, if your mind says, "You're gonna fail!" you wouldn't get into an argument with it. Instead, you would simply notice what it's doing as a habit of your mind and then decide whether you want to listen to it in a given moment. There are lots of different ways to do this, and chapter 2 will introduce you to a bunch of techniques.

Willingness. Willingness means showing up to what hurts inside of you with openness, care, and compassion—and without dwelling in it. It involves treating your painful thoughts and feelings as invited guests, rather than sworn enemies.

Sounds like acceptance, doesn't it? Willingness is another term for acceptance. But remember, "acceptance" doesn't mean that you like the thing you're accepting, or that you're giving up on making changes in your life. Rather, it means showing up to circumstances that give rise to painful thoughts and feelings with openness, making an impact where you can, and letting go of what you can't control. Chapter 3 is all about willingness.

Present moment awareness. Present moment awareness means connecting to what's going on right now through our senses, rather than through the constant narration of our minds. It's a necessary part of processes like defusion and willingness, but it is also an important process in and of itself. Think of what it's like to walk into a beautiful, verdant garden on a sunny day. Outside of what your mind might say about the experience (e.g., "Wow, this is beautiful"), there is the experience itself, available through your five senses: the smell of the flowers, the constellations of shapes and colors, the feeling of sunlight on your face, the warmth of the air against your skin, the chirping of birds, the chittering of insects, the sound of your feet making contact with the dirt, and maybe, if you're lucky, the taste of a ripe strawberry, straight from the ground. Present moment awareness means bringing that kind of focus—deliberate yet flexible attention—to all of your experience, from the delightful stuff, like that strawberry, to the difficult stuff, like your anxiety or sadness.

Values and committed action. These two processes are so intimately connected that we put them together. In ACT, a "value" is a way of being, a choice about how you want to *behave* on an ongoing basis, no matter what is showing up inside you. ACT encourages you to articulate your values and then commit to actions that serve those values. For example, even when things are tough and frustration is bubbling up inside of you, you can still choose to be kind, curious, and patient *in your actions*. "Kind," "curious," and "patient" are values words, so if these words capture your values, you can choose specific actions to take in the service of those values—and you can commit to taking those actions with openness to and curiosity about whatever may result.

Flexible perspective taking. Flexible perspective taking means cultivating a sense of self that is bigger than what you experience inside of yourself—thoughts, feelings, sensations, memories, etc. It means taking the perspective that thoughts and feelings will come and go, but *you*—as the being who's experiencing these thoughts and feelings as they arise and pass—are always here, and you are not your thoughts and feelings. They are simply part of you, and a temporary part at that.

You are also not your stories about who you are: "I'm not as smart as these people, but I'm smarter than those," "I'm a child of alcoholics," "I mess up every relationship I'm in," "People don't understand me," and on and on. Flexible perspective taking makes it possible to take a lot of other useful perspectives, like putting yourself in the shoes of someone else or imagining an older, wiser you looking back on your life right now.

Of course, this can get kind of heady, so we do a lot of work in chapter 6 to help you experience this perspective. Like most ACT stuff, you can't really understand flexible perspective taking until you *do* it.

Finally, though not explicitly part of the ACT model, we've added a section on *positive psychology*, a set of techniques, practices, and routines based on the science of happiness, flourishing, and living meaningfully, which we think fits perfectly with ACT. Positive psychology was developed by researchers who thought, "Maybe we can put some of our focus not only on relieving suffering, but also on enhancing people's lives." It's not about replacing pain with pleasure or negativity with positivity. Instead, it's learning to turn our focus to what's delightful, meaningful, or awe-inspiring when it's there, so that we don't miss out on the great stuff that life has to offer. Chapter 7 is all about that.

How to Use This Book

This book is a workbook, meaning there are lots and lots of exercises sprinkled throughout the text to help make the concepts come to life. And ACT itself is an experiential model of behavior change and personal growth. What that means is that most of the concepts need to be *experienced*, not just talked about. For example, it's one thing to say that control can be problematic and then cite a little research. It's another to give you an opportunity to really map out how control operates in your life, how well it works, and what the costs are.

There will be lots of exercises like the one you've done so far, and there will be others too: thought experiments, metaphors to consider, goofy but instructive things to do with your hands and your body, mindfulness exercises and visualizations, and concrete skills to practice and actions to take in your life outside of this book. These exercises will help make the concepts become real in your life. It's one thing to talk about acceptance. It's another thing to actually practice, in the moment, mindfully making space for shame or embarrassment as it emerges in your body, and reminding yourself to be kind to it, all while focusing on being the person you want to be, no matter the circumstances. That takes practice!

What we know about skills-based therapies like ACT, as well as self-help books in general, is that the way to really get the most benefit out of them is to actually do the exercises. So, we encourage you to do as many of the exercises as you can.

That being said, we've also built *The ACT Skills Workbook* to be used flexibly. First, it's modular, meaning that each chapter is an independent module, and you can work on the chapters in any order. After reading this chapter, where we introduced you to some basic concepts, you can jump to any chapter that catches your eye.

Is your inner critic making your life a living hell? Go straight to the chapters on defusion (chapters 2 and 7). Is most of your headspace taken up by thoughts about the past or future, so much so that you miss out on what's going on right now? Check out present moment awareness (chapter 3). Are you already struggling to figure out what we mean by values, or do you hold so rigidly to the values you have that they are confining you? Check out the section on values and committed action (chapter 5). When a painful feeling like sadness or shame shows up, do you go running for the hills? Turn straight to willingness (chapter 4). Do you want to look at what you can enhance in your life right away, like gratitude, awe, and moments of pleasure? Go to take a look at positive psychology skills (chapter 8).

Of course, none of the principles in these modules are wholly independent of the others. They are meant to work synergistically. When we teach ACT to therapists, and when we do ACT in a structured way with our clients, we do so in roughly the same order as the chapters of this book. For example, willingness is often a hard place to start. So, doing some of the defusion and present moment awareness work ahead of time could make it a little bit easier. We encourage you to jump around if you like—and to get the full benefit, it's probably important to spend time with each chapter and read each one to the end.

Learning to Notice

A couple of pages ago, shortly after we asked you to map out the way control works in the short and long term, we invited you to do some reflecting. We are going to do that *a lot* in this book. We would argue that one of the most important muscles to build in doing ACT work is your noticing muscle. That's because most of us humans—including the two people writing this book—spend most of life on autopilot. We rarely stop and think much about why we are doing what we're doing and what its impact is going to be. The first step in doing things differently is to learn to notice. So, we'll invite you to notice over and over again. You might just get sick of the word "notice"!

Challenging Yourself and Knowing Your Limits

We encourage you to really put your heart into this work, to deeply consider the questions we ask and take meaningful risks in your life. That could mean anything from doing something bold that you have been avoiding for fear of failure to doing an exercise that intentionally brings you closer to do some kind of pain in your life—a memory, a sadness, a worry, or some other psychological pressure point.

At the same time, we encourage you to take care of yourself. You don't have to push yourself to be the best at this. There's no best. There's no perfection. There's no way to "get it right." There's only lots of practice. And you don't have to do anything you're not ready for or not willing to do. So, for example, if we ask you to pause and practice mindfully breathing in and out through a painful emotion—as we do in chapter 4, on practicing willingness—you get to choose when you do it, what emotion you choose to do it with, and, ultimately, whether you do it at all. Your growth toward living well doesn't require you to do every exercise in this book. What we want for you to get out of this book is a new orientation toward your thoughts and feelings, and a new focus on living a life that's meaningful for you. And there are many different paths to achieving that.

Who We Are

We're both licensed mental health professionals who specialize in ACT. Matt is a social worker, meaning he has a master's in social work, and he's been practicing psychotherapy for nearly twenty-five years. He's been teaching others to practice psychotherapy, especially ACT, since about 2008. He's an instructor in psychiatry at a medical school, and he works with students studying medicine, nursing, and similar professions every day to help them navigate depression, stress, and anxiety. Jen is a psychologist, meaning she has a PhD in psychology, and she's a professor of psychology at a university, where she does research, teaches psychology classes, and mentors budding psychologists. As a therapist, she specializes in helping people cope with cancer and end of life. She's been doing ACT since its early days, when she was an undergraduate working in the psychology lab of Steve Hayes, one of the cofounders of ACT.

Both of us have published multiple books and academic papers on ACT and ACT- related subjects. Both of us regularly train and consult with professionals on how to implement ACT. It's safe to say that we live and breathe ACT every day, both in our work and also in our personal lives. All the exercises in this book are exercises that we have done with ourselves as well as the people we serve. We are excited about ACT not just because we see it make a difference for people in our offices every day, but also because it's made an enormous difference in our own lives.

Thus, we've written the book in a fairly personal way. We will refer to ourselves from time to time and give examples from our own lives. This is important to us: the ACT model suggests that we all struggle in similar ways, whether we are helpers or the people being helped. We all fall into habits of unnecessary control, and we all fall into letting go of things that are meaningful when we are not paying attention. So, we are speaking from personal as well as professional experience.

The Science of ACT

Will this book help you? The honest answer is that we don't know. Self-help books tend to make lofty claims. But very few self-help books are researched to show whether or not those claims are true. This book has not been subjected to research—at least not yet. We both have a deep respect for science, so we're not going to make any claims we can't back up.

However, we wouldn't write this book if we weren't confident that it could make some kind of difference. ACT has been researched in over one thousand well-designed studies ("randomized controlled trials," for you nerds out there). It has also been shown to make a difference for an impressive array of problems, from stress and burnout to anxiety and depression to quitting smoking and coping with cancer. Studies have even shown it helps with severe and persistent mental illness, like schizophrenia (Jansen et al. 2020). Though there's always still work to be done, it has been shown that ACT can make a difference in many different cultural contexts, not just among well-educated, predominantly white North Americans and Western Europeans (ACBS n.d.; Musanje et al. 2023). It's even been researched by the World Health Organization (WHO) as a self-help intervention for helping refugees cope with the stress of displacement during wartime (Acarturk et al. 2022).

And ACT is not just a model for psychotherapy, though that's where it started; it's also been adapted into workshops, apps, coaching, parent training, and, yes, self-help books. And in all these forms, the science has shown that it can make a difference. (We've included a list of some self-help books that have been researched and shown to be effective in the back of this book. Feel free to check them out.)

Getting Professional Help

Some ACT self-help books have been shown to help reduce clinical problems like depression and anxiety (e.g., Muto, Hayes, and Jeffcoat 2011; Ritzert et al. 2016). That being said, we don't think a self-help book is sufficient for every problem. If you work through some of this book, and you discover that it's not really making a difference, you might benefit from seeing a mental health professional. If you're really struggling right now, you might just start there. If you already have a counselor or therapist (we use those words interchangeably), you can ask them whether you can work through the book as part of your treatment, if you like. If you're in a crisis, call or text 988 in the United States to reach the 988 Suicide and Crisis Lifeline, 24/7. Finally, if you're having thoughts of suicide, we recommend you get support right away. No one needs to deal with that stuff alone.

Okay, now that you know how to use this book and have a sense of what it's going to be about, let's get back to ACT.

CHAPTER 2

Defusion

You Are in Charge, Not Your Mind

If you are going to reduce unnecessary avoidance and control in your life, and get more connected to your values, the first barrier you encounter may be your own mind. The minute you start consciously moving toward something that is important, something that might elicit anxiety or fear of failure, your mind might say, "Wait, do you really want to do this? What if it hurts? I bet there's another way. In fact, I don't think you're really capable of doing this. Maybe you should keep thinking about it for a little while before doing anything."

This is a feature, not a bug. Our minds are built to protect us from harm. As we noted in the introduction, early humans on the African savanna had one primary objective: stay alive. To do this, they need to eat, procreate, stay connected to their group, and protect themselves from threats. Therefore, having a world-class threat detector (i.e., their mind) was the key to staying alive and propagating the species. That's what some scientists think accounts for our *negativity bias*—the tendency of our minds to focus more on the bad stuff than on the good stuff.

But what worked hundreds of thousands of years ago doesn't completely work for life in the twenty-first century. Our minds continue to look out for threats when there are rarely any (literal) threats nearby. There are generally no lions, tigers, and bears in our immediate environment, and most of us—though sadly not all of us—have enough to eat, people to love, and communities to connect to.

So, even when we are having the best of times, our minds might say, "What if I don't feel this way tomorrow?" Even when we are surrounded by people we admire, our minds might say, "I hope they don't discover all of my flaws." And even when we are falling in love, our minds might say, "Watch out. This could hurt." Meanwhile, we may miss out on the beauty and vitality in our work, play, and relationships.

Defusion

So, what can we do about this? Can we turn our minds off? Sadly, the answer is no. Decades of research suggests that trying to push thoughts away ultimately makes them more persistent (Wegner 1994). Remember: If we asked you not to think of a white bear for the next thirty seconds, what would happen? More white bears! But we *can* learn a new way to relate to our minds, one that limits the power of their misapplied threat detecting. This is called defusion.

EXERCISE: An Experiential Introduction to Defusion

Rather than just telling you about defusion, it's better if we show you first. Then we can explain things a little bit.

To do this exercise, pick a thought that tends to get really sticky for you. By sticky, we mean a thought that shows up when things are hard, sticks around for a long time, and tends to make things harder. Don't pick the hardest one, but pick something that you tend to overfocus on or one that encourages you to stay away from important things in your life. It could be something like these:

"God, my brother drives me crazy when he rants about this."

"My colleague is so self-absorbed."

"Why am I so anxious all the time?"

Do you have a thought? If it involves a lot of words or ideas, see if you can distill it into something specific like the thoughts above. Minds don't always offer us discrete sentences, but it's helpful to narrow down the chatter into a distinct message if there is one.

(By the way, this exercise can be powerful. But it does have risks, like any other exercise in this book. It might elicit some uncomfortable feelings. So, you're welcome to stop at any point. At the same time, we encourage you to consider continuing with the exercise while you just notice those uncomfortable feelings and see what happens.)

Now write your thought the space below, just like those thoughts above.

"_____"

Take a look at these words and imagine that they are not just words, but a physical manifestation of your thought. By some miracle, you have been able to remove it from your mind and stick it right in front of yourself to look at. Look at it again from this perspective. This is *you* looking at *your thought* the way you might look at it in your mind.

Now, if doing that doesn't make sense, that's okay. Just do the exercise as best you can without thinking about it too hard.

Now say the thought to yourself silently and preface it with the words "I'm having the thought…" In other words, say "I'm having the thought…" and then follow it with your thought.

After you do it, don't think about it too hard—just notice what that's like for a moment before continuing to the next sentence.

Now do the same thing, but use the words "My mind is saying…." In other words, say "My mind is saying…" and then follow it with your thought.

Notice what that's like before going on to the next sentence.

Notice that we are just getting a little bit of linguistic distance here. We are just noticing we are having thoughts.

Next, check in with yourself and notice if this thought is familiar to you. Does it have a *history*? Has it been showing up for a while? How far does back does it go? Has the same message shown up throughout your life but with different words? Spend about fifteen seconds considering this.

Now, check in with yourself again and notice whether this thought is *habitual*. Does it tend to show up in specific situations, or in many situations that are like each other in some way? Or does it just show up all the time? Spend about fifteen seconds considering this.

Now, ask yourself how *useful* the thought is. Where in your life does it help you? Where in your life might it get in the way? Is it the right tool for a particular job, or is it like a hammer when what you really need is a screwdriver? Spend about fifteen seconds considering this.

Now, look up at the sky, either directly above you or through a window, and imagine that the thought is up there in the distance, floating in the clouds. Really imagine it. (If you can't see a window where you are, use the ceiling.) Don't try to make it float away. Just notice it floating there, perhaps drifting gently across the sky. Do this for about fifteen seconds.

And finally, just go back and take a look at that thought you wrote.

Reflection: Before we debrief about the exercise, write a little bit about the experience. What did you notice?

_____

_____

_____

_____

_____

_____

If the only thing you wrote was "But my thought is still there!" take a moment to think about what else besides the thought might be different. Are *you* different in some way? Are you relating to the thought differently in any way?

The Impact of Defusion

I (Matt) have done this exercise a bazillion times in my therapy groups and my ACT workshops, both for professionals and for the public. Here are the kind of things people typically say:

"It feels lighter."

"I feel like it isn't so important anymore."

"I don't feel so stressed out by it."

"At first, the thought seemed even more powerful, but then over time, it felt more like just a thought."

Was your experience at all like these? Not everyone has the same experience. It's totally okay if none of these things happened for you. But here's our goal when we practice defusion: Treating thoughts as what they are—just thoughts. Not facts. Not truths. Not evidence of our character. Just the products of a habitual word machine that spins stories out of our daily experiences.

Think about it: we have so many thoughts all day long, and most of them we hardly pay attention to: "What can I have for lunch?" "That guy's driving like a doofus." "Mm, another cup of coffee sounds good." Few of these thoughts get sticky for us. They just come and go.

The difference between the really powerful, sticky thoughts that make your life hard and all the other thoughts that just pop into your mind is not the thoughts themselves. Instead, it's how you are relating to them.

When a difficult thought shows up, we typically relate to it like it's something we have to contend with. I (Matt) often have to deal with some version of "I'm not doing enough," "I should be doing this differently," or "I'm doing it wrong." This doesn't just happen once in a while. This shows up *constantly*, bubbling under the surface.

When I am at my best in terms of relating to these thoughts—and you can be sure that I'm not always at my best—I treat them as just something that is passing through my mind, a mental habit that I don't really need to listen to or do anything about. I'm perfectly capable of tying my shoes, making my breakfast, and moving through my workday without giving any credence to these thoughts.

That doesn't mean that these thoughts are not painful. They're actually pretty painful sometimes—painful and exhausting. But the less power I give them, the less effect they have over me, and often, the less they stick around.

Let's go back to the last exercise for a second. Notice we didn't do anything to try to make the thought change or go away. We didn't argue with it. We didn't reason with it. We didn't try to find more truthful thoughts to respond to it with. We simply practiced relating to it in a variety of new and sometimes playful ways to start developing a new relationship with it. One in which it's not your enemy—it's simply a thought.

From this perspective, a few things become possible:

We can decide whether the thought works for us in the current situation. In other words, we can decide whether it's useful information we need to act on.

We can follow a different path if necessary, one that might be guided by something else—like our values (see chapter 6)—instead of what the thought might typically lead to, like procrastinating, getting into arguments, or criticizing ourselves.

Let's go more deeply into some of the basic ways of practicing defusion you tried in the previous exercise.

Basic Defusion Skills
NOTICING YOUR THOUGHTS

The first skill in defusion—and really the first skill in almost every psychology strategy that involves responding to thoughts more effectively—is noticing exactly what it is you are thinking. It means turning your attention to your mind and seeing what's there. Let's get some practice.

EXERCISE: What Do You Notice?

Set a timer for sixty seconds. Watch your mind the way you would watch cars going by, and every time something shows up, write it down on one of the lines below. This could include specific thoughts (e.g., "Where is this going?"), images (e.g., a picture of you sitting down to lunch later), or memories (e.g., a memory of the conversation you had with your child earlier in the day).

Thought: _____

Thought: _____

Thought: _____

Thought: _____

Thought: _____

Thought: _____

Thought: _____

Thought: _____

Thought: _____

Thought: _____

Thought: _____

Thought: _____

What did you notice? Was it some combination of words, sentences, and memories? Did you have distinct thoughts, or were they all jumbled up, bumping into one another? If this exercise is tricky for you to do, that's okay. Don't overthink it (no pun intended); just keep going with these exercises and it will become easier over time.

"I'M HAVING THE THOUGHT…"

One of the simplest ways to defuse from thoughts—and often the most effective—is to repeat what your mind is saying, but preface it with something that will give you some distance. For example, you could think "My mind is saying…" or "My brain tells me…" or "I'm having the thought…" Putting these words before your thoughts as you notice them helps you see them as simply thoughts.

Let's say this is what shows up in your mind: "I really hate shopping for groceries; I freeze up with every decision I have to make." Instead of responding the way we might typically respond, such as agreeing with the thought (e.g., "Yeah, it sucks") or challenging it (e.g., "You don't have to hate shopping—it would be easier if you made a list ahead of time"), you would instead do something like the following:

"I'm having the thought 'I really hate shopping for groceries, and making decisions makes me freeze up.'"

That's all.

The exact wording doesn't matter. What counts is using a little bit of language to give you some separation from the thought without agreeing with it, arguing with it, or trying to push it away.

EXERCISE: "I'm Having the Thought"

Take a moment to practice. Set a timer for sixty seconds, and every time a thought arises in your mind, repeat it back to yourself while prefacing it with "I'm having the thought..." or "My mind is saying..." You might benefit from writing these statements down in the space provided the first time you try it, but you don't have to.

_____

_____

_____

_____

_____

_____

_____

NAMING YOUR STORIES

You'll likely notice your mind tends to offer you similar kinds of thoughts in similar situations (and if you have a mind, it probably does). Naming your stories is about looking for the overarching theme, or "story," your mind typically tells.

For example, maybe your mind doesn't just wrestle with grocery shopping, but also wrestles with any daily task that isn't especially pleasurable, like taking out the trash or doing the dishes. You might say something like:

"My mind is telling me the 'I hate doing this because it's tedious' story again."

Or, if your mind typically stresses about the way you will feel when you do something—for example, that you will feel bored, tired, or burdened—you could say:

"There's the 'this is going to suck' story again."

By using the word "story," we don't necessarily mean the thought is not true. The thought could be true, false, or unknowable. Most defusion strategies just focus on what is happening in your mind, not whether it's true or not.

You don't have to use the word "story" if you don't want to. You could call it a "narrative" or "meme" or something else. It's simply a label for the typical themes your mind offers you.

EXERCISE: Identify Your Stories

It can be helpful to identify a bunch of thoughts that show up in particular situations to find the common theme. For example:

Situations	Thoughts	What's the story?
I'm working under a tight deadline.	"I should have started sooner." "I can't believe my boss has such unreasonable expectations." "I hate that I have to do this."	The "it shouldn't be this way" story.
I'm talking to someone who I think is more successful than I am.	"I'm not as good as them." "I bet they didn't really work for what they have." "What can I do to be like them?"	The "comparing myself to other people" story.
My partner is upset with me for something I didn't do around the house.	"Don't they know I'm busy?" "Why are they so demanding?" "How can they be upset? They didn't do that thing I asked them to do, either!"	The "I'm right, they're wrong" story.

Give it a try.

Make a list of stories your mind typically tells you and where they tend to show up in your life. Don't worry about getting *all* the stories down or getting them just right. We're just trying to strengthen the muscle of noticing, so it doesn't have to be perfect. (And, by the way, it will never be perfect!)

Situations	Thoughts	What's the story?

EXAMINING WORKABILITY

Remember "workability" from chapter 1? Just like we use workability in ACT to determine whether a behavior works for our lives, we can use it to decide whether a thought is worth listening to. When a sticky thought shows up, ask yourself the following questions:

How workable is this thought for *what's going on in this moment?*

How workable is it for *living the life I want to live?*

Here's an example: Naya is baking cookies in preparation for her daughter Pratheepa's birthday party later that day. Whenever she is hosting a gathering at her house, even if it's just for little kids, she gets nervous and starts ruminating about how well she will do: "Will Pratheepa like it?" "Will the other parents think I have done enough?" "Is the house clean enough?" Because she has begun to notice how her mind works, she has given this familiar series of thoughts a name: "the inadequate parent" story.

After noticing the story, she might say to herself, "Is this story workable?" She might observe that it's adding to the nervousness she already feels and that focusing on it makes her less focused on what she's doing. So, it's not really workable for *what's going on in the moment.*

And if she steps back and looks at the big picture of her life, she might observe that this story typically takes her away from being the mom and the host she wants to be. She knows from experience that giving too much power to this story leads to her being irritable with Pratheepa and not really paying attention to her guests. Also, there's a mom who's coming whom she'd like to get to know a little bit better. So, it's not really workable for *living the life she wants to live.*

It might sound like workability is in either/or proposition. But it doesn't have to be. Some sticky thoughts *do* tend to work for us in some situations. And usually, if they are habitual, they have certainly worked in the past.

Let's go back to Naya. Looking back on her life, she knows that the inadequate parent story is part of a long-standing pattern of comparing herself to other people and judging herself as falling short. It's something she learned by example from her parents, who were immigrants to the US, faced a lot of hurdles, and were understandably very focused on succeeding. Comparing themselves—and their daughter—to other people was a good way to know what was possible and how they were doing. They passed on this habit out of love—it motivated them and helped them build a life they were proud of in a new place.

Naya recognizes it was a useful motivator—it got her going and led to a lot of success in school, extracurriculars, and friendships. But she realizes now that it has consequences. In situations like this, she's extra nervous, and it's hard for her to enjoy the moment, because she's always preoccupied with whether or not she what she's doing it right—whatever "it" is.

At this point in her life, when she's working on being present for her family and savoring meaningful moments, she knows that this story is not so workable anymore. She has realized that "being present" and "savoring meaningful moments" is motivation enough to devote herself fully to putting together a memorable party for Pratheepa. The story doesn't stop showing up throughout the day, but she continues to just make note of it and make space for the anxiety that accompanies it. And she puts her energy into being more present, especially in the beautiful moment when her daughter blows out the candles on her cake.

Let's get some practice looking at the workability of what your mind offers you.

EXERCISE: Exploring the Workability of Your Thoughts

Think back over the recent past—go back a few weeks or so—and recall some situations where your mind got really sticky. Identify what was showing up in your mind and how workable it was. (This exercise, along with several others in this book, is available in worksheet form at http://www.newharbinger.com/53738.)

Situation	Thoughts or stories	How workable was listening to your mind for what was going on in the moment? For living the life you want to live?

It's worth pointing out—again—that we are not encouraging you to condemn these thoughts as "bad" or "negative" or "distorted." We are taking a very practical approach: thoughts are going to show up, they serve a purpose, and sometimes they outlive their purpose and lead to unintended consequences.

Take a moment to check in: what are you noticing right now as you do these exercises? Are you noticing some relief or a sense of freedom from these thoughts? Are you noticing some uncomfortable feeling show up—sadness, embarrassment, or something else? That's okay: there's no right way for you to respond. If you're feeling something uncomfortable, see if you can make space for that feeling without trying to push it away. Sometimes getting close to our thoughts can stir up some pain. We can fall into judging ourselves for things we don't have any control over. We can see ourselves as defective in some way. You are not defective if you have an inner critic, negative patterns of thinking, or any kind of unworkable thought. You're human. See if you can just make space for whatever is showing up, and then take the next action in your life. That could mean taking a break from these exercises for a little while or continuing on to the next one.

Take the Next Meaningful Action

Mindfully noticing that you are thinking—whether through observing, getting a little linguistic distance, or naming your stories—is typically the first step in defusion. Asking whether your thought is workable might be the second step—but it doesn't have to be. There is no perfect sequence, just lots of useful options.

But sometimes, just noticing is a little insufficient. After all, not only is the thought still there, which you often can't help, but it's very sticky, knocking around in your mind and absorbing your focus despite you stepping back from it.

What could you do next? There's really no requirement to *do anything*. But we are "doing" sorts of animals, so it's helpful to have something in your back pocket for that tricky moment when you've noticed your thought, but you don't know what comes next.

Let's go back to some of those sticky thoughts and stories. Again, pick a thought that tends to show up and make life hard, one that you are willing to spend a little time with for the next few moments:

Thought: _____

Now, let's consider where this thought typically leads. Though thoughts don't cause our actions, they certainly have an influence on us. And some sticky thoughts are reliably followed by certain kinds of behaviors. For example, a thought like "What if I fail" might be followed by procrastination and worrying. A thought like "I can't believe she left the dishes out when I asked her five times to put them away" might be reliably followed by irritable sniping at your partner. Or a thought like "My child isn't happy; I must be a bad mother" might be reliably followed by checking out, perhaps by scrolling through social media or drinking alcohol to numb the pain.

So, where does this thought typically lead you? What kind of behaviors typically show up when your thought shows up?

_____

_____

_____

_____

_____

_____

_____

If you notice yourself writing about behaviors you are not especially proud of, you're not alone. Most of us have some kind of pattern like this. If looking at these behaviors kicks up more sticky thoughts, do your best to just notice those thoughts without giving them much energy. If you're judging yourself, know that the compassionate—and frankly more effective—response is more like what we're doing here: teasing out the patterns of your thinking and decoupling those thoughts from your actions, so that you can make choices that work better for your life.

So, what would work better for your life? What could you do the next time this thought shows up that might be a little bit more aligned with being the person you want to be? With living the life you want to live?

For example, let's go back to the thoughts from a few paragraphs ago, and think about what some more workable actions might be. You might have the thought "What if I fail" and keep working on a task. You might have the thought "I can't believe she left the dishes out again" and commit to yourself to have a civil conversation later, once you've cooled down. Or you might have the thought "I'm a bad mother" and notice, with kindness, that it tends to arise in your mind when your kids are having normal human emotions, and then talk with your child about what they're feeling without trying to solve the problem for them.

What could you do differently the next time the sticky thought you chose shows up? Think about specific behaviors that work better for your life:

_____

_____

_____

_____

_____

_____

_____

_____

_____

_____

EXERCISE: Bringing It All Together

Over the next few days, you might experiment with bringing these strategies together using the worksheet on the next page. Get some practice, and then when you feel ready, move on to the next section, where we add to this skill set with some additional defusion tools.

Situation	Thoughts	What was their impact on my behavior?	How workable was listening to them for what was going on in the moment? For living the life I want to live?	If I had not listened to them, what might I have done differently?

More Defusion Skills

What you've done so far is the basics: noticing, naming, and examining the impact and workability of your thoughts. You might be thinking, "This really isn't doing anything—I'm still having lots of negative thoughts." Of course you are. As we noted before, your mind is built to focus on negative things. From the ACT perspective, the problem is not that you have negative thoughts, but rather how you relate and respond to them. When negative thoughts come, do you treat them as literal truths, meaningful evaluations of the world, or evidence of a greater likelihood that bad things will happen? Or do you notice them as what they are: tools you can choose to pick up or not.

Keep this in mind as we introduce you to some additional ways to practice defusion.

REPEATING THOUGHTS

One of the coolest studies by ACT researchers was run by Akihiko Masuda and his colleagues in the early 2000s (Masuda et al. 2004). They wanted to see if a defusion technique, one that had been around since long before "defusion" was even a word, would make the difference they thought it did. This technique was described by English psychologist Edward B. Titchner in the early twentieth century. He claimed that when a word is said out loud over and over, it loses its literal meaning. In other words, it just becomes a bunch of sounds.

In the study, participants were asked to identify some negative thoughts they had, like "I'm dumb," and practice different ways of responding to them. There were three types of possible responses: defusion, thought control, and distraction. In the defusion response, participants repeated a word the way Titchner described. They distilled their thought to a single word (e.g., dumb) and then said it quickly for thirty seconds. For thought control, participants were encouraged to do anything they wanted to, such as positive self-talk, positive imagery, or deep breathing. Finally, the distraction technique was reading about Japan.

The participants rated both the believability and the discomfort associated with each thought both before and after each technique. Defusion reduced the believability and discomfort the most. What the researchers also found was that just telling participants about defusion didn't have any impact at all on the believability and discomfort related to the thoughts. That's interesting: it suggests that you have to *do* defusion to benefit from it, not just talk about it or explain it. Which is what we're about to do here: have you *experience* it.

Let's try it with the next two exercises.

EXERCISE: Repeating a Neutral Word

It can be helpful to start with a neutral word. Take a look at the word below:

Milk

Let your mind imagine what this word represents. What do you see? Hear? Smell? Taste? Let it be as real for you as you can.

Now, set a timer for thirty seconds, and repeat the word quickly out loud to yourself.

All done?

Before we talk about the exercise, write down what you noticed:

_____

_____

_____

_____

_____

_____

People typically notice that all those experiences your mind creates—the images, the sounds, the smells, and the taste—begin to dissolve and are replaced by something very physical. Specifically, the feeling in your mouth associated with the effort to say the word repeatedly, and the odd, evolving sound of each spoken word butting up against the next. Before you started repeating the word, it might have felt a bit like some milk was actually right in front of you. And then after repeating it, it was no longer there. Yet the word "milk" is not something that we've tried to get away from. We've actually spent a lot of time with it.

EXERCISE: Repeating a Negative Thought

Now let's try the same exercise with a thought you have that tends to get in your way. It can be the same thought you've used in the previous exercises, or it can be a different thought entirely—whether it's a judgment (e.g., "I'm not enough"), a worry (e.g., "what if I fail?"), or something else. Pick one thought you're willing to spend a few moments with.

Thought: _____

If you're willing, take a look at the thought for a moment and allow it to affect you in the way it typically affects you.

Next, rate how believable it seems in this moment and how much discomfort you are feeling on a 100-point scale, with 100 being the highest believability or discomfort:

Believability (0–100): _____   Discomfort (0–100): _____

Now, grab your timer again and say it out loud quickly, over and over, for thirty seconds.

Rate the thought again now that you've done the exercise:

Believability (0–100): _____   Discomfort (0–100): _____

Reflect a bit on the exercise. What happened? Try to focus on the actual experience of it—physically, sonically, and otherwise.

_____

_____

_____

_____

_____

_____

Did this thought do the same thing that "milk" did? Did you notice the believability and discomfort changing in some way?

Often, those numbers go down the way they did in the study. Sometimes, however, they don't. Whatever happened, you are not doing it wrong. We are simply trying out different strategies, and those strategies are not going to have the same impact on everyone. Some will work for you more than others.

Breaking Your Rules

Early humans needed to develop rules for living: if it's dark out, you shouldn't stray from the campfire because you might get eaten; you should always make use of the entire animal you kill because there might not be another one for a long time; you should always look after the people in your group, because we depend on each other for survival.

Contemporary humans have rules as well—lots and lots of them. Some of them are explicit, like the ones we tell our kids: "Don't go out into the cold without a coat on," "Look both ways before crossing the street," and "Share your toys with your brother." Some of them are less explicit, but equally powerful: "If I show my anger, I'm a bad person," "I should always be prepared and on time," "I shouldn't feel anxious, because that means I'm weak," or "I shouldn't feel sad anymore because it's been six months since my mother died."

Whether explicit or implicit, we don't walk around thinking very hard about them. But we live them out, whether or not we are aware of it. Think of a rule like, "If I show my anger, I'm a bad person." This one shows up among the people we work with as therapists quite a lot, especially among women who may have been raised to be polite and who were scolded or shamed when they revealed that they were angry. Their early training as children, and the multitude of experiences they've had around anger since then have powerfully shaped this rule into something that they live out. And when they break the rule, they feel ashamed and guilty, often without really understanding why.

Think about how a rule like this can get you into trouble. Sometimes anger is called for. Sometimes you need to get your child's attention before they walk into traffic. Sometimes you need to advocate for yourself when others are not treating you well. Expressing anger doesn't need to involve shouting, kicking, and screaming. Without anger, a lot of important work in the world would go undone. It's a motivator for instigating social change. Think about the civil rights movement or the movement to reduce greenhouse gas emissions. Anger is necessary! So, if you have a rule about anger, sometimes it might be worth breaking it.

In this next exercise, you are invited to uncover some of your rules with a series of prompts. Notice the frequency of words like "should" and "always" in the prompts, as well as consequences like "being a bad person." Rigid rules often have that kind of flavor. For each prompt, just write the first thing that comes to your mind, even if it sounds ridiculous, even if your logical mind knows better. If one doesn't resonate with you, feel free to skip it.

EXERCISE: Uncovering Your Rules

I should _____

Everyone should _____

I should never _____

I should always _____

I should feel _____

I shouldn't feel _____

I always have to be _____

I should be the kind of person who _____

I'm not the kind of person who _____

If I don't _____, then I have failed.

If I _____, then I have failed.

If I don't _____, then I'm a bad person.

If you are a good person, you should always _____

If you are a good person, you should never _____

To be acceptable, I need to _____

To be loved, I need to _____

To be happy, I have to _____

I have to _____, otherwise _____

Other rule: _____

Other rule: _____

Other rule: _____

Now that you've listed a few rules, let's take a look at how they operate in your life. In the next exercise, we will put your rules to the workability test. (First, we'll show you an example of the exercise based on the kinds of rules some people we know—inside and outside of our offices—struggle with.)

EXERCISE: Exploring the Workability of Your Rules

Rule	Workability: what are the benefits of following this rule?	Workability: what are the costs of following this rule?	How could you break this rule when doing so could reduce your suffering or help you build a richer life?
I should always be kind to people.	It helps me build relationships with other people. I feel good about myself.	I often don't speak up for myself, and when I finally do, I'm already so angry that I come across as harsh.	I could work on speaking up sooner while still being kind. I might not get so resentful.
I should always feel grateful for everything I have.	I'm good at recognizing the good things in my life.	I feel guilty when I don't feel grateful, and I wonder what's wrong with me.	I could allow myself to feel what I feel while also recognizing there are good things in life that are sometimes hard to feel good about.
I shouldn't feel anxious in social situations—there's nothing to be scared of.	It helps me push through my anxiety when I'm meeting new people.	I feel bad about myself for feeling anxious and it's still there.	I could give myself permission to feel anxious even though I don't like it. It won't stop me from engaging with other people.
If I get mad at my kids and occasionally don't want to be around them, that makes me a bad mother.	I try my best to be understanding, no matter what they do—not going to bed on time, not cleaning their rooms, fighting with each other.	I constantly have a low-grade sense that I'm a bad mother, because though I love them, I have a lot of complicated feelings when they are misbehaving.	I could treat my irritation and frustration as normal and totally compatible with loving them and being a good (enough) mother.

Rule	Workability: what are the benefits of following this rule?	Workability: what are the costs of following this rule?	How could you break this rule when doing so could reduce your suffering or help you build a richer life?

You probably noticed that most of your rules work in some way. We wouldn't have them if they didn't ever serve us, whether at some time early in our life or right now in the present. The problem isn't that we have these rules—everyone does. The problem is when these rules become fixed, rigid, and unbreakable—when it feels like not living them out will lead to dire consequences. And we live out those rules even when they're not working for us. We follow a rule like "Don't ever say an unkind word" even when it leads to getting our feet stepped on. We follow a rule like "Always do your best" even when it leads to driving ourselves into the ground with overwork. So, keep paying attention to your rules and experiment with breaking them.

Facing Worry with Action

Everyone worries. We all know what it's like to get wrapped up in repetitive thoughts about things that could occur in the future that we have little control over. And it can be pretty miserable, especially if we are prone to worrying a lot. So why do we do it? Again, think of early humans. The ones who worried about bad outcomes—who prepared for famine, or who assumed that the eyes glowing in the dark were attached to a lion, not a friendly stranger from the next valley—were more likely to stay safe. It's likely we descended from humans who were natural worriers. If we didn't worry, we might not have survived. But as with most things rattling around the minds of contemporary humans, the things we worry about now are not life-threatening. They are often just uncomfortable and potentially stressful. Worry is an understandable response, but often not a very functional one.

Worry can be contrasted with *active problem solving*—identifying a problem and taking steps to address it. Worry can *feel* like problem solving, which is probably one of the reasons why we do it—we get a sense that we are doing something when our mind is busy, busy, busy. And occasionally, we arrive at something meaningful, which gives us a little bit of a reward and probably makes it more likely that we will worry again. Think of a slot machine: you may pull it one hundred times and get nothing. But if you get a jackpot the one hundred and first time you pull the lever, then you may be motivated to keep pulling again, even if you don't get anything for the next two hundred, three hundred, or four hundred pulls. You keep going, hoping for that jackpot.

One of the best ways to suck the power out of worry is to identify small, concrete actions you can take, and then take them. When you take action, especially action related to what you are worrying about, you give your mind something to chew on instead of spinning its wheels. Here's an example.

I (Matt) give a lot of presentations: I train mental health professionals on ACT in multiday workshops. I've given talks on stress, sleep, and mental health stigma at big-name tech companies. And in my current day job at a university counseling center, I regularly talk to groups of students about stress, coping, and resilience. With all this practice, I'm not especially nervous when I give a presentation. It just comes naturally… sometimes.

Sometimes I get nervous for no reason I can identify, and worry starts to bubble up in anticipation of giving a talk. Recently I was giving a talk the medical students who were about to embark on four to six weeks of dedicated study time—basically doing nothing else—in anticipation of their first board exam. The exam is called "Step 1," and my presentation was called "Step 1 Can't Eat You." Great title, right? I compared the stress of this high-stakes test to the stress of facing a lion who is intent on eating you. I offered them a few of the skills in this book, reminding them that though it may feel like there is a lion chasing them, the lion is really in their mind. It's a great talk, so what was I worried about? I was worrying that they would be bored and restless, ready to get moving on studying, not sitting through yet another mandatory lecture about practicing self-care.

Here's a little secret about me: your boredom is my kryptonite. As a lifelong ham and attention-seeker, the best way to destroy me is to look uninterested. According to my worried mind, I was going to spend an hour trying to capture the attention of bunch of people who just wanted to get on to the next thing.

But I know a few things about coping with worry. So, I made a plan—a concrete series of steps to take that would hopefully diminish the power of the worry, even if those steps didn't make it go away. So, I made a slide for the section on coping with worry in my presentation that looked like this:

Facing Worry with Action

Worry	Is what I'm worrying about in my immediate control?	What can I control? What are the concrete actions I can take to respond to this worry?
I've got a presentation to give. What if no one finds it interesting?	Not really. They will find it interesting or they won't.	Set aside sixty minutes to update old slides. Revise the section on worry. Get to the office early so I don't feel rushed. Get a fancy coffee on the way to work for comfort.

Notice how little control I had over the thing I was worrying about—their boredom. There's no way that I could guarantee some students wouldn't be bored with my talk. But I could take small, concrete actions that were related to what I was worrying about. Getting busy and taking concrete action occupied my mind and my hands with meaningful activity, which left less room for worry.

So, the next time you're worrying, try the same thing with the worksheet on the next page.

EXERCISE: Facing Worry with Action

Worry	Is what I'm worrying about in my immediate control?	What can I control? What are the concrete actions I can take to respond to this worry?

Summing It Up

The mind is powerful, but not so powerful that it has to be in charge. When there is an opportunity to try to control your thoughts and feelings—to stop them from pulling you away from what's meaningful—*you* get to be in charge, not your mind. That's easier said than done, however. These exercises, based on the principle of defusion, can help you get a little distance from your mind, so that it doesn't feel so believable, so truthful, so commanding. Your mind won't stop offering you suggestions, worries, predictions, criticisms, and on and on. But you can live alongside it and learn to listen more deeply to the important stuff—the stuff that tells you about real danger (when it's there) and the stuff that articulates your values. More skills for doing this follow in the rest of the book.

CHAPTER 3

Present Moment Awareness

Living with Your Eyes Open

Welcome to the present moment. It's kind of lovely here. When we wake up from the fog of living inside our thoughts and notice the moment we're in, we can experience some cool stuff. We can also better back away from our difficult thoughts and feelings, and then move toward our most important values. The present moment is pretty amazing.

Rather than being in the present moment, we often operate from inside our stories and ongoing narratives, and don't really experience the world around us. Inside our heads, we focus on experiences we've had in the past and things we worry will happen in the future—so much so that we often miss what is happening here in the present. We are way too busy thinking about our experiences to actually experience them.

Take the example of Susanna. When Susanna has a conflict with her partner, she is often angry for days, and it takes a long time for her to recover and address the conflict. This is because she spends so much time circling over and over in her thoughts about the conflict—chiefly about who was right and who was wrong—and she has little awareness of what her actual thoughts and feelings are. She isn't aware of how she is responding or the consequences in her environment, because she's so busy replaying the conflict and reacting to her thoughts about it.

ACT has a lot to offer Susanna, but before it can be helpful for her, she needs some skills for noticing the moment she's in and seeing what is happening while it's unfolding. Only then can she notice her actual experiences, back up from her difficult thoughts and feelings, and move in the direction of her most important values.

As we talked about in chapter 2, from an ACT perspective, the content of thoughts and feelings isn't the problem. Rather, it is *seeing the world through* those thoughts and feelings and letting them direct our lives that causes us to feel like we need to avoid or control them. In order to step out of that cycle, the first thing we need to do is notice: (1) what we're thinking, and (2) the fact that those thoughts are guiding our behavior in unworkable ways. To do that, we need some present moment awareness.

Noticing the Present Moment

What exactly do we mean by "the present moment"? How could we be in any place other than the present moment? Aren't we always in the present?

When we talk about the "present," what we're actually talking about is paying attention to something besides our mind's constant chatter. We come in to the present moment, which involves noticing where we are, what we're doing, and even what we're thinking. The exercise below will give you a first taste of what we mean.

EXERCISE: Thoughts, Feelings, and Sensations, Here and Now

We are thinking, feeling, and sensing all the time, but since we often aren't aware of these private experiences, we often mindlessly react to them. A big goal in ACT is to increase our awareness of our thoughts, feelings, and sensations as they occur, so we can increase our ability to flexibly respond to them.

One way to step out of autopilot is to slow down and purposefully come back to your actual experience in the moment. For example, in this moment, as you are reading this, what is your actual experience? As I (Jen) write these lines, I notice that my lower back is a little sore, that my right ear itches, and that the spots where my feet are touching the floor are a tiny bit numb. I notice that I am having thoughts about what is on my schedule for today, and I notice that when I think about the tasks of the day, I feel a slight pressure in my chest. When I really explore the pressure in my chest, I notice that my shoulders are a little tense and I have feelings of excitement, anticipation, and stress about my day ahead.

Your turn: tune in to the actual experience you are having right now, in terms of body sensations, thoughts, and feelings. See if you can notice what is happening here and now, and write it down below.

_____

_____

_____

_____

_____

_____

_____

Taking a minute to notice how our experiences, as they occur, allow us to back up from our thoughts and automatic reactions, as well as increase our awareness of what is occurring minute to minute. We can purposefully practice "building the muscle" of being more able to notice by closing our eyes and systematically focusing on what we notice.

EXERCISE: Just NOTICE

This exercise is designed to help you purposefully practice paying attention to things around you and return to the experiences you are having in the moment, as they occur. The following practice (along with some of the other meditation exercises throughout this book) is available as a guided audio file via http://www.newharbinger.com/53738. You can listen to the audio track or read the instructions below and practice on your own.

If you decide to try it on your own, you can use the acronym "NOTICE" to prompt your attention to the important aspects of the exercise.

Notice:

- What sounds you can hear around you (**N**oises)

- What the air feels like on your skin (**O**xygen)

- What thoughts are floating around in your head (**T**houghts)

- What you feel or notice in your body (**I**nsides)

- Who you're with or who is around you (**C**ompany)

- What is in the world around you (**E**nvironment).

Whether you use the audio file or give it a go on your own using the following text, you can jot down the things you notice in the space provided.

EXERCISE: Noticing Practice

To begin, sit in your chair in a way that allows you to be aware and awake, but not rigid or tense. You can either close your eyes gently or pick a spot in front of you and let your gaze rest there softly. Whatever works best for you.

Begin by turning your attention to your breath, noticing the rising and falling in your chest and belly as you breathe in and breathe out. Follow your breath from the tip of your nose to the bottom of your lungs and back out again. There's no need to try to control your breath in any way. As best you can, just let your breath be natural. But if you find yourself controlling it a little bit, as we sometimes do, don't fight that. Just notice.

Now, turning your attention from inside of you to outside of you, tune in to the sounds of the room you're in. Notice the variety of sounds across the landscape of your hearing. Notice how each sound occupies its own place in that landscape.

Now, turning from outside to inside, gently direct your attention to the places where your body makes contact with your chair or whatever surface you're making contact with. Tune in to the sensations of touch or pressure there.

As we do this exercise, you'll inevitably notice your thoughts or mind grabbing your attention and pulling you away. When this happens, you're not doing it wrong; your mind is just doing what minds do. When this happens, just notice and then turn your attention gently back to the moment—without a fight, without judging your mind.

Now, moving from inside to outside again, open your eyes, look around, and take in all the shapes, colors, and textures around you. See if you can tune in to something that you hadn't noticed recently—or perhaps ever.

And now closing your eyes, if they were closed before, or keeping them open if that's your preference, turn your attention back to where we started: watching your breath as you breathe in and out. And follow with two or three more breaths in this way, and then let go of the practice.

In this exercise, you might have noticed lots of things, or you might have noticed it was really hard to notice anything. Anything is great. Remember that the goal is just to practice noticing. Make notes about what you noticed below.

Noises: _____

Oxygen (breath): _____

Thoughts (mind): _____

Insides: _____

Company: _____

Environment: _____

General things you noticed from trying this exercise:

_____

_____

_____

_____

_____

_____

_____

EXERCISE: Logging Your Noticings

Over the next week or so, practice closing your eyes and either listening to the audio file or doing this exercise your own. At the end of each day, complete a brief log about what you noticed when you returned to the present and what the practice was like.

Day	Observations

Being able to stop what you're doing and be in the present is the first step to being able to use present moment awareness to respond differently to your thoughts and feelings. It is an important skill. And—bonus—always available to you for the low, low price of free!

That said, present moment awareness is not a one-time-and-you've-got-it skill. You might have experienced some lovely peacefulness or calm when you did the exercise above, and that is great. You also might have noticed that your mind jumped all over the place and it was difficult to stay in the present very long—that is also great. Consistently practicing coming back to the present moment, over and over again, is what allows us to notice our thoughts and feelings and move in the direction of our values. We can think of this as training our minds to not get caught up in our thinking. And it's likely your mind will need some training for you to be able to use it when you most need it.

Mindfulness

One skill that can assist in this training is mindfulness. Mindfulness can be defined as "paying attention to the present moment, with curiosity and kindness, on purpose and without judgment" (Kabat-Zinn 1994). In other words, noticing. Mindfulness is a common way to practice present moment awareness, and while it can be useful in itself, in ACT we use it as a tool for staying flexible in how we respond to our difficult thoughts and feelings.

Sometimes people struggle with mindfulness—it can feel a little intimidating and complicated at first. When we first talk about mindfulness, people often worry that they are "doing it wrong." It is not uncommon for someone to sit down for a session of mindfulness meditation and spend the whole time lost in thoughts about whether they are meditating correctly. The trick is just to notice these thoughts (as thoughts) just as you notice everything else. Ultimately, as long as you are noticing, you are doing it correctly. (Even if what you're noticing is the thought that you're doing it incorrectly!)

Noticing Without Judgment

As noted above, a key element of mindfulness is noticing what we are experiencing with curiosity and kindness—and *without* judgment. This can be especially difficult to do when we are lost inside our thoughts about something. We often can't even notice that we are judging, because we are so hooked by the thoughts that we don't notice the distinction between the judgment and the thing we are judging.

EXERCISE: Observe and Describe

In this exercise, you will practice observing your experiences and then describing those experiences both judgmentally and nonjudgmentally. This will help make the distinction clearer and strengthen your ability to notice the difference between judging and just noticing. You can do the exercise with the instructions that follow or with the guided meditation audio file at http://www.newharbinger.com/53738.

Start by looking around you where you are right now. Notice what you see. What objects are around you? What color are the walls? What types of furniture are in the room? What patterns do you notice?

Now try to purposefully apply a judgment to something that you see. Maybe you see an "ugly" lamp or a "beautiful" table. Can you notice the difference between the evaluation and the plain description? Write an example of each in the "visual" row in the table below.

Now try the same task with sounds you notice. What sounds can you hear around you? First, describe the sounds with descriptive language, and then apply a judgment to highlight the difference. Maybe you can notice a fan humming and can see that your mind calls it an "irritating" or a "soothing" hum. Write what you notice in the "auditory" row below.

Now notice what you smell. Is there an odor around you? Notice what it is, and then see what the evaluative or judgmental description would be. Write it in the "smell" section of the following table.

Finally, notice your body. What sensations can you notice? Again, notice the sensation in plain language and then apply a judgment or evaluation to the sensation to see the difference. Maybe you notice a tightness in your back or neck. See what judgment your mind wants to apply to that sensation and write it in the "body" section below.

Object/Experience/Sensation	Judgment
Example: Sound of a light humming, sound is slightly variable when I listen carefully, even though it sounds uniform	Annoying humming sound
Visual:	
Auditory:	
Smell:	
Body:	
Other:	

Noticing judgment can be a good way to build our awareness of the world around us, while preventing us from getting caught by our thoughts. Try to practice noticing when your thoughts are colored by judgment, and see if you can help yourself describe things more objectively.

The exercise below is another brief mindfulness exercise designed to help you bring mindful awareness to all of the things going on in the present—your body, your breath, your thoughts—while letting go of judgments. Again, you can access a guided version of this same meditation practice at http://www.newharbinger.com/53738, or read the section below and follow the instructions.

EXERCISE: Brief Mindfulness Practice

Begin by sitting comfortably with your feet flat on the floor and your back supported by your chair. Arrange your head, neck, and shoulders so that they are upright but not stiff. You may either close your eyes or, if you prefer, leave them open with your eyelids half-closed and your gaze directed at a point approximately thirty degrees in front of you. This is not the only way to practice mindfulness, but it's a useful way to start.

In your mind's eye, turn your attention to your breathing. Observe the rising and falling of your breath in your chest and belly. Follow your breath from the tip of your nose to the bottom of your lungs and back out again. Though you will likely be tempted to, there is no need to try to control your breathing in any way. As best you can, allow your breath to breathe itself.

Next, turn your attention to your body in the chair. Scan your body, observing the places where you make contact with the chair. Notice the sensations of touch or pressure there.

As you do this exercise, you will notice that your mind tends to drift off. This is completely normal; it's what minds do. Minds rarely stop moving, and they can usually be found problem solving, predicting, worrying, planning, remembering, and judging. When you notice that you have drifted off, gently bring yourself back to the present moment.

Now, turn your attention to your feet inside your shoes. Notice the varieties of sensations there: touch, pressure, temperature. See if you can pick out each individual toe. If it helps, wiggle your toes a little bit. Next, turn your attention to the places where your skin makes contact with the air: on your face, on your hands, wherever. Notice the sensations there. Now, turn your attention to the sounds around you. Sounds both inside the room and, if you can pick them out, outside the room.

Finally, bring your attention back to your breathing. Watching the rising and falling in your chest and belly as your breath flows in and flows out. Allowing it to be as you gently observe.

This is mindfulness: paying attention to the unfolding of experience without judging and without trying to change anything. You can bring this quality to any experience. You need not practice formally as we have done today, but practice can help you to be mindful when it really counts: when you work, when you play, and when you engage with others.

Now, let's bring this exercise to an end. Simply observe one or two more breaths, open your eyes if they are closed, and silently congratulate yourself.

When you have finished this mindfulness meditation practice, write down what you noticed for your future reference. What happened? What was the experience like for you?

_____

_____

_____

_____

_____

_____

_____

_____

_____

Mindfulness practice can be very useful when we're feeling overwhelmed, or for increasing our awareness of what we are experiencing moment by moment. Again, there is no "wrong" content to notice and no "wrong" way to notice—whatever comes up, we can notice it.

Building Mindfulness Informally

While sitting in mindful meditation can be very useful to build skills for present moment awareness, it should be noted that sitting still with closed eyes is not for everybody. Luckily, meditation is not the only way to build mindful awareness of the present moment. Anything we do that allows us to "wake up" to the moment we're in can build mindfulness and present moment awareness. Below are two exercises that allow you to practice the skill of waking up without sitting down to meditate.

EXERCISE: And Now I'm...

One reason mindfulness meditation is a helpful practice for people is that they literally stop everything else and just concentrate on one thing—noticing. When you meditate, the goal is to breathe and know you are breathing, have thoughts and know you are thinking, have sensations and know you are having sensations. The goal isn't to not have experiences, but rather to know you are having them as an observer.

In this exercise, we will try to amplify this awareness. This involves naming what you are doing, out loud if you can, as you do it. Speaking aloud forces us to notice each element—without taking shortcuts. Here is a brief example of what this might sound like:

"Okay, I'm noticing a little soreness in my elbow, and now I'm noticing that I'm wondering why my elbow would be sore. I'm now noticing the feel of my feet in my shoes. Now I'm noticing that the clock says 5:05, and now noticing that when I saw the time, my stomach muscles contracted slightly, and I'm noticing that I'm having a worry that I might be late if I don't leave soon."

Give it a try now, as you write in this workbook. Notice what you're doing and feeling, out loud, right now, and write your noticings here:

And now I'm noticing…

_____

_____

_____

_____

_____

_____

_____

EXERCISE: Daily Noticing

Now, try to bring this capacity to other activities you find yourself doing over the next week or so. You can write your process or speak it out loud anytime to help yourself be more grounded in the present moment. Write down what you notice in the table below. Of course, if you do the exercise out loud, you may need to make sure nobody is around, or they may become a little concerned about you!

Day	Observations

EXERCISE: Mindfulness of Daily Activities

In addition to dictating internal experiences out loud, another way to increase our present moment awareness and ability to step outside of thoughts, feelings, and sensations is to purposefully pay attention—just like you do during sitting meditation—to the everyday activities that make up your life. You can brush your teeth with awareness, wash the dishes with awareness, or eat a sandwich with awareness—just about any regular activity can be turned into a mindfulness activity.

The trick with informal mindfulness practice is to pick an activity that you are intentionally going to try to do mindfully and then practice that each time you do the activity. For instance, each time I (Jen) load my dishwasher, I intentionally try to focus on the feel of the water running over my hands as I rinse the dishes. I notice the sounds that the dishes make when I set them in the dishwasher, and I notice the sensation of how each wet dish feels in my hand as I move it from the sink and place it in the dishwasher rack. Again, the goal here is just to take yourself off autopilot and step out of the constant chatter of your mind to pay full, nonjudgmental attention to the task that you're engaged in.

For this exercise, pick an activity that you do frequently, and try to bring mindful awareness to the entire task. When your mind wanders, which it will, just bring your attention back to the task. If you get through the whole task without being present, that's okay, just notice where your mind went and try again the next time you do the task. Use the space below to note your experience.

What was the task you chose, and how did it go? What did you notice?

_____

_____

_____

_____

_____

_____

_____

_____

Summing It Up

This chapter is focused on building skills for noticing the present moment, rather than acting—or reacting—in our environments while caught up in our thoughts and feelings. This can be difficult to do consistently, so you'll probably need to be extra patient with yourself. As you develop more and more present moment awareness, you will find that it will become easier to pause for a minute and stay grounded in the face of difficult emotions and situations.

However, in these skills and all the other ones taught in this book, it is important to remember that the goal is not perfection; it is effort. There is no outcome that we should be concerned with. Rather, you're engaged in a *process* of moving toward your values and how you want to show up in your life. And in this process, commitment to practicing your skills is what's important, not the permanent achievement of some perfect state. That means you will often "catch yourself" completely forgetting about the present moment. Each time you notice this, just notice that you notice it. As long as you're noticing, you're doing the work.

CHAPTER 4

Willingness

Opening Up to Whatever Shows Up

The ultimate goal of ACT is to give you different ways to respond to difficult thoughts and feelings—other than avoidance—so that you can move toward your most meaningful values. One key new way to respond to difficult experiences is with *willingness*. Willingness is a tricky concept in ACT, but in essence it involves intentionally letting difficult emotions and experiences be present when it's better to do so in the long run. Let's unpack what that means.

The More Good, Less Bad Mindset

As we mentioned in chapter 1, we humans have a strong bias toward having things go a certain way in our lives. We have a built-in, reflexive tendency to try to grasp as hard as we can on to positive experiences and to push away negative ones. We're not even usually aware when we do this. If we see an object we want, we move toward it. And if we encounter something we don't like, we move away.

Despite being hard-wired to do this push and pull, it often backfires on us. Over time, "good" things become less good, they end, or they are out of reach. "Bad" things tend to come along no matter how hard we try to prevent them. And the more we try not to feel things like anxiety, loneliness, discomfort, or vulnerability, the more we tend to feel just that (remember the white bear idea from chapter 1).

Nonetheless, we persistently hold on to attempts to have "more good" and "less bad." This is particularly the case when we have really big or scary emotions. Think of a time you were really overwhelmed by fear, grief, sadness, or pain. What did you feel, physically and emotionally?

_____

_____

_____

_____

_____

And what did you do?

_____

You probably felt like nothing was as important as managing that feeling so you could get things back to normal. And you probably tried the things we usually try in these situations—fleeing from whatever caused the feeling, avoiding it, or trying desperately to "fix" the feeling and make it go away. The bigger the emotion, the more we lose our ability to respond in any other way than to try to control it. When our systems are overloaded, our focus becomes narrow and the only option that feels available to us is to shrink the uncomfortable feelings as quickly as we can.

EXERCISE: Your Go-To Control Strategies

In ACT, before we can do something different in the face of difficult emotions, we need to first identify our own unique control strategies. As we talked about in chapter 1, control strategies are any behaviors we use to avoid, minimize, suppress, or manage unwanted thoughts, feelings, bodily sensations, and experiences. Control strategies are not always bad or problematic, but we often engage in them without even noticing, so it's useful to explore them.

Here's an example from Jen's life:

Even though it is a big value of mine to do so, I have always had a hard time asking people for what I need to be different in my relationships. When I have to make a specific request that I think might be uncomfortable or inconvenient for the person I'm requesting it from, I have lots of worries, anxious thoughts, and physiological stress before I even begin speaking. I worry that they will get upset or that my request is unreasonable, even when I know logically that it's not. I spend a lot of time overpreparing and practicing what I want to say to reduce these worries. And before the discussion, I ruminate on all the ways things could go wrong to feel less vulnerable if they occur. During the discussion, I am so focused on getting it out that sometimes I end up being sharper than I mean to be.

Think about your own life. Are there areas where you notice this more good/less bad happening? If so, what are your go-to strategies for controlling?

Place where I am stuck	Unwanted feelings	Control behavior
Jen's example: Asking for what I need	Thoughts that something could go wrong Vulnerability Fear, psychological and physiological	Overpreparing Practicing a lot Worrying/Ruminating Focusing on finishing
Your example:		
Your example:		
Your example:		

We all have go-to control strategies, especially for very difficult thoughts and feelings, and for the areas in our lives where it feels most important. In fact, sometimes when it feels like there is a lot on the line, our control strategies (and difficult thoughts and feelings) get even bigger.

An Alternative to Control: Willingness

As mentioned above, "willingness" in ACT refers to the behavior of being open and receptive to difficult, painful, or unwanted thoughts and feelings, in order to have a meaningful life full of the things you care about. This might involve being open to feeling afraid or anxious, experiencing grief or sadness, or having unwanted thoughts or memories. It may even include being open to feeling physical pain or uncomfortable body sensations.

EXERCISE: Personal Willingness Goals

Think about the control strategies you listed in the last table. What experiences were those strategies intended to help you control? Take a look at the list below, and put a checkmark by any of the willingness situations that you find difficult in your own life.

- ☐ Being willing to be vulnerable in relationships
- ☐ Being willing to face things I fear
- ☐ Being willing to sit with boredom or lack of distraction
- ☐ Being willing to face mistakes I've made in the past
- ☐ Being willing to let people care for me
- ☐ Being willing to receive negative feedback
- ☐ Being willing to trust others
- ☐ Being willing to forgive myself or others
- ☐ Being willing to make big changes in my life
- ☐ Being willing to have difficult conversations
- ☐ Being willing to feel lonely

In the space below, try to write down the specific feelings or emotions you might have to be willing to feel in each situation you checkmarked. For instance, if you were willing to trust others, what emotions might you have to navigate?

_____

_____

_____

_____

_____

_____

_____

Finding Purpose Alongside Pain

In this section, we will illustrate the connection between difficult thoughts and feelings, and the things you find most meaningful in life. To start with, we will do a little free writing about something you care about.

EXERCISE: Two Hands

In the space below, write about some part of your life that's very important to you, something that gives your life richness and meaning. It could be your relationships with family and friends, your spiritual life, your creative practice, or the work you do every day. What is it about this part of your life that makes it so special to you? Really paint a picture.

Here's an example from Matt's life:

A part of my life that's very important to me is the work I do to train therapists, coaches, and other helping professionals in acceptance and commitment therapy. It gives my life richness and meaning because I get to help other professionals develop skills that will not only make a difference in the lives of people they serve but also—if I'm lucky—in their own lives as well. One of my favorite parts of being an ACT trainer is occasionally hearing from people that my training workshop marked a turning point in their career, one in which they started approaching the people they serve differently.

Brief summary: Training others in ACT

Write about your own example below:

_____

_____

_____

_____

_____

_____

_____

_____

_____

Brief summary: _____

Now think about some pain you experience in this area of your life—some combination of thoughts and feelings that can show up inside you and get in the way of this part of your life. Maybe it's an irritation, an anxiety, or a sadness. Maybe it's a worry that you're not good enough. Whatever it is, it's something inside you that can get in the way of what you really care about. If the thoughts and feelings relate to something someone else in your life does, like a friend letting you down, identify what shows up inside you in response to that, like sadness or anger. After you've written about it a bit, summarize it with a few simple words.

Here's an example from Matt's life:

No matter how much I prepare, I always have moments during the training when I realize I'm criticizing myself for something. There's a little part of me that's always evaluating everything I do, and it can criticize me for just about everything: being too much of a show-off, not caring enough, talking too much, getting too intellectual, and on and on and on. It can lead me to feeling anxious and a little bit ashamed, even if I know I haven't done anything wrong.

Brief summary: My inner critic

Write about your own example below:

_____

_____

_____

_____

_____

_____

_____

_____

Brief summary: _____

Now that you have articulated this stuff, we'll show you something about the relationship between this valued part of your life and the difficult thoughts and feelings that show up when you're engaged with it.

To start with, hold up your hands in front of you, with your palms facing up. Space them about a foot apart.

Imagine that in your left hand you could hold that part of your life that is really meaningful to you, that part that brings you such richness and vitality. As odd as it may seem, imagine that you are holding it right there in front of you. Make it real and feel the weight of it there as you hold it.

And in your right hand, imagine that you could hold that pain, that combination of thoughts and feelings that shows up and gets in the way sometimes.

While you're holding your hands up like this for the next minute or so, we'd like to tell you about something extraordinary.

Through the miracle of data science and algorithms, we have created a secret technology to remove the pain you are holding in your right hand. And we're going to introduce it to you!

Here's the secret: all you have to do is bring that hand down by your side. But don't do it yet!

Before you do anything, we have to tell you about the side effects. There are always side effects, right?

In order to remove that pain, you're going to have to remove that thing you care about as well. Don't do it yet, but to bring down your right hand—the one with the pain in it—you also have to bring down your left hand.

Let's just pause here for a moment before we do anything. Don't think too hard—just sit with the implications. Is this a deal you want to make?

Okay. If you're willing to make that deal with the universe, then on the count of three, drop both of your hands. If you're willing to make that deal, when we get to "three," you'll drop your hands.

Ready? Here we go.

One… two… three.

What did you notice? _____

_____

_____

This exercise is meant to define what we mean when we talk about willingness—we are often asked to hold tremendous pain in order to live our most important values. Now let's talk about specific ways to do that.

Willingness and Values

As you noticed with the Two Hands Exercise above, willingness and values are intricately connected in ACT. When we talk about willingness, it is never for just the sake of being willing, but rather for the sake of having an awesome life with the things you care most about.

When you imagine your future self living a life that feels meaningful to you, what do you see? Maybe you picture yourself in a close, connected romantic relationship. This, of course, requires you to be *willing* to be vulnerable with a partner or to be *willing* to possibly have a broken heart along the way. Maybe you picture yourself finding a job that would be more authentic for you, and you would need to be *willing* to risk a change to stable circumstances to pursue that job, or *willing* to feel insecure or make mistakes as you learn a new role.

EXERCISE: Values-Based Willingness Behaviors

A few exercises ago, you identified your go-to control strategies. Now it is time to talk about what to try instead in those situations where you find yourself stuck, using your values as a guide to help you be *willing*.

In Jen's example above, there was a lot of focus on what was uncomfortable about asking for what she needs, but not the why. Here is the rest:

> *While asking for what I need is rough for me, it is also connected to some of my most deeply held values. I value being clear and non-resentful in my relationships, and I value not making myself smaller than I am. I value being as gentle and understanding of others' points of view as I can, and also trying to give myself that same kindness and fairness. I value taking good, proactive care of my relationships. I try to push myself to ask for what I need, even when it's uncomfortable, so I don't accidentally get grumpy with people just because they didn't do something for me that I didn't even ask for.*

In the following table, write down the places you're stuck, your unwanted feelings, the control behaviors you engage in to manage those feelings, the values you hope to bring to each stuck place, and the willingness behaviors you might try out to live by those values, rather than giving in to the need to control your experience.

Place where I am stuck	Unwanted feelings	Control behaviors	Relevant values	Willingness behavior
Jen's example: Asking for what I need	Thoughts that something could go wrong Vulnerability Fear, psychological and physiological	Overpreparing Practicing a lot Worrying/ruminating	Being clear and non-resentful Not making myself smaller Being kind and fair to myself Not being reactive or grumpy	Figuring out what I need Giving myself equal care Clearly asking for what I need
Your example:				

Place where I am stuck	Unwanted feelings	Control behaviors	Relevant values	Willingness behavior
Your example:				
Your example:				

Now that we have begun narrowing in on the ways willingness might be relevant to you, let's define both willingness and control in a more physical way. This classic ACT exercise and metaphor has multiple origins, but is probably most closely tied to an exercise in a chapter Matt wrote in 2014 (Boone 2013), with echoes from exercises and metaphors existing throughout the ACT literature (e.g., Harris 2008; Hayes et al. 1999).

EXERCISE: Butterfly Exercise

This is called the Butterfly Exercise, but you won't know why until the very end. To begin, take a small piece of paper and write down a thought or feeling you struggle with. It doesn't have to be the most difficult thing you experience, but make it something you genuinely struggle with. Any thought, feeling, memory, or body sensation will work.

Once you have written the unwanted experience on the piece of paper, imagine that the feeling is somehow embodied in the paper—that the paper actually *is* the feeling somehow.

Now, with the words facing toward you, try to push the paper down into the table as though you are trying to push it away from you. Push it gently at first, and then really try to get it away from you. Notice what that's like in your body.

Now notice, is it gone?

Next, hold the piece of paper between your two hands and squeeze your hands together as hard as you can without hurting yourself. Notice again what that feels like in your body.

And notice again, is it gone?

Finally, hold your hand open, palm up. With the other hand, gently drop the paper into your own hand and catch it like it's a butterfly landing on your hand. See if you can hold it gently, like something precious. Now bring it in close to your body, as though it is not your enemy but rather something you could take care of.

Now look around you and see what you see in your environment. And look back at what you have in your hand.

Close your eyes and hear what you can hear around you. And look back down at what you are holding.

Now notice, is it gone?

Notice if there is a difference between the various ways of touching the paper. Notice what feels different between the different ways you relate to the paper, even if the paper and its content stay the same.

Use the space below to jot down your thoughts and reactions, as well as things you noticed while doing this exercise.

_____

_____

_____

_____

_____

_____

This exercise gives a physical example of what we mean when we talk about willingness—rather than using energy and effort to push away difficult thoughts, feelings, and experiences, we can change our response to them.

Willingness Is Not Wantingness

Being willing to experience an emotion is not the same thing as wanting to experience that emotion. Willingness emphasizes the ability to accept and sometimes even embrace emotions, thoughts, and bodily sensations that we might absolutely not want, because doing so is in the service of our values. For example, you might very much dislike being emotionally vulnerable, but you might be willing to do so when you must ask for what you need in a close relationship. You do not need to want to be vulnerable to be willing to do it. Or, you may not want critical feedback on a project, but you might be willing to ask for it in order to improve the project or your work in the long term. Ultimately, being willing to experience difficult emotions is a behavior, a choice. You can be willing to experience difficult emotions whether you want to or not.

Willingness often happens in stages. The first stage is primarily about taking action related to our values. In subsequent stages, though, willingness may include the act of purposefully building our capacity to accept difficult emotions when they come up, in order to not automatically avoid them in the future.

SLOW DOWN, HOLD STEADY, WELCOME IT ALL

While we talk about willingness as an important response for when we're having difficult experiences, in reality, willingness often looks like doing an awful lot of nothing. Simply letting our existing emotions be there, without fighting them, is also willingness. This is especially the case when our normal, automatic response is to try to avoid them. Just hanging out with them and letting them be there can sometimes be a totally new experience.

When emotions come up, it can sometimes be helpful to have a structured way to practice willingness. To do this, people sometimes use the acronym NAIL to help remember what to do.

EXERCISE: NAILing It

We should note that we didn't come up with this technique, and different therapists and meditation teachers talk about it as slightly different variations (RAIN, RAIL, RAFT), which all have the same general purpose.

Here are the steps:

Step 1. Notice

The first task is to notice that you are having a feeling. This sounds basic, but you'd be surprised at how long we often have difficult thoughts, emotions, or experiences before we even realize that they are present. Remember, noticing doesn't involve solving, eliminating, rationalizing, talking ourselves out of, or avoiding. It just involves noticing that an experience is there.

Step 2. Allow

Once we have noticed that we are having a thought, emotion, or experience, the next step is to purposefully not push it away. This means not doing something to reduce it, like trying to rationalize it or think of something else, distracting yourself, or fighting with the experience. Allowing is the slightly passive experience of just resting with it and not doing anything.

Step 3. Investigate

The next step is to investigate. This piece has two elements. First, investigate the story your mind gives you about the experience. What thoughts are there? Does the story involve any "shoulds" or "shouldn'ts"? Try to just curiously investigate the story without getting wrapped up in it or talking yourself out of it.

Second, investigate what you feel in your body. Explore what sensations are there, and how you feel this particular experience physically. What do you notice about the sensation? Is it heavy? Light? Tight? Loose? Hot? Cool? Whichever sensations are there, just notice them.

Step 4. Let It Be

The final step is to let the experience be right where it is, without changing it or trying to control it. Even if it is uncomfortable, see what happens if you let it be just as it is. Sometimes the feeling will be gone by the time you get to this step, sometimes it won't. Either way, just gently set it down (without pushing it away), and return to your life a little bit stronger for having purposefully practiced a little willingness.

If you like, you can use the space below to jot down your thoughts and reactions, as well as things you noticed while doing this exercise.

_____

_____

_____

_____

_____

_____

If you'd further practice opening up to emotions in this way, try the Mindfulness of Emotions exercise in the online additional materials, or start with the more basic mindfulness exercises in chapter 3.

Where Control Works

Although controlling thoughts and feelings doesn't always work out, there are parts of our experience that we can more easily control. First, let's clarify what we mean by "control." When we talk about control, we mean *directly* control, the way you might control the light in the room by flipping a light switch or the way you might control whether the floor is clean by sweeping the floor. That's just not possible with thoughts or feelings. If a thought or feeling shows up, it shows up. We can't just flip a switch and make it go away.

But we can control what we do—the actions we take and where we put our energy and attention. To illustrate this, take a look at the table below. On the left is what we can't directly control; on the right is what we can.

What you can't control	What you can control
• Spontaneous thoughts (e.g., "I'll never be good enough") • Spontaneous feelings (e.g., a sense of anxiety or sadness) • Spontaneous sensations (e.g., elevated heart rate, a pit in your stomach) • Other people's thoughts and feelings • Other people's behavior • Your past • Your future	• What you do with your hands, your feet, and your voice—i.e., your actions, what you *do* • How you *respond* to your thoughts and feelings—e.g., whether you criticize yourself or just notice them without fighting them • What you make important in your life—i.e., your values

Notice again that the things we often try to control are not really in our control:

Thoughts, feelings, and sensations. Thoughts, feelings, and sensations will arise continuously throughout the day. They are part of the operations of our brain and body, and they show up because of the complex interaction of our genetics, our epigenetics (experiences that make specific genes express themselves), our life history, and our current situation. They are the result of the perfect storm of all these factors (and more), and they are not your fault—or evidence of a character defect.

Other people. We also can't control other people. They will do what they do. They will also think and feel what they think and feel. We can have some influence on other people, to be sure, but ultimately, they are out of our control.

The past. The past has already happened. Ruminating on what could have been doesn't get us anywhere, though it's very compelling. Who wouldn't want to change the past? But we really can't. It's obvious, but despite that, many of us are trying to mentally undo painful moments in the past by thinking about them repeatedly.

The future. We also can't control the future. Again, we can have an *influence* on the future. We can do everything we can to make the future turn out in a particular way for ourselves and the people we love. But we cannot guarantee that the future will be what we want it to be, no matter what we do. It's just out of our control.

But we *can* control the stuff in the righthand column, and focusing there can make an enormous difference in our lives: what we do, how we respond to our thoughts and feelings, and what we make important in our lives.

What we do. No matter what we're feeling—excitement, anxiety, happiness, shame, sadness, delight, boredom, whatever—we can usually move our hands and feet and use our voices, assuming those parts of our bodies work as directed. Which is to say, we can *act*, and the way we act doesn't have to perfectly match the way we feel; we can shape our actions in a way we can't always shape what we feel.

All of us can think back to experiences in which we felt one thing but did another. If our mind tells us we are "not good enough," we can actively act as if that's not true. (Also, what on earth does "not good enough" mean? There's no such thing as a "good-o-meter" that measures our goodness. This is just a subjective, usually biased, story our mind is telling based on a limited amount of information. And "good enough" is a goal that keeps moving just out of our reach. More on that in chapters 2 and 8!)

Similarly, if you're in a situation that makes you nervous—say, you must have a tough conversation with someone you love—and a feeling of anxiety arises, you can acknowledge that feeling of anxiety while you behave as bravely and kindly as you can.

How we respond to thoughts and feelings. We can also develop skills for responding in new, more workable ways to our thoughts and feelings. That's a big part of what this book is about—stay tuned.

What we value. And, ultimately, we get to choose what we make important in our life. For example, when we are feeling frustrated with a family member, friend, or colleague who is driving us crazy, we can choose whether we are guided by something that might get us in trouble, like the thought, "I'm going to tell them how full of sh*t they are" or something bigger, like a conscious choice to be understanding yet assertive. We get to choose this, and we can practice living it out, even when our thoughts and feelings are pulling us in the opposite direction. This is an example of living by our values, and values are a big part of ACT.

Summing It Up

Humans are control machines. We try to control everything in our worlds, including our feelings. This is such an automatic response that we usually don't even notice we're doing it. In this chapter, we built skills for noticing when we try to control our emotions, exploring the cost of attempting to control them, and trying out new ways to deal with our difficult feelings—rather than bringing down the hammer in a bid to squash them.

The goal in ACT is to live a more meaningful, values-driven life. A key part of doing that is making room for the full range of emotions we experience as human beings, including experiences that are uncomfortable, unwanted, or distressing. Rather than creating a narrow focus that reduces our negative experiences to *bad* and *unwanted*, willingness leads us to a broader focus that helps us see the valued directions into which we can move, if we're willing to experience even tough emotions in the service of what matters.

CHAPTER 5

Values and Commitment

Powerfully Connecting Behavior to Values

An essential element for living an amazing life is thinking about *how* we want to live that life. This is the opposite of behaving in the fixed, automatic ways we adopt in order to control our experience. Focusing on reducing negative emotions leaves little room for thinking about what we would want our life to look like if managing those feelings wasn't our top priority.

In chapter 1, we asked you to imagine that in your left hand, you held all the things that are most meaningful and bring the most vitality to your life. And in your right hand, you held all the feelings you struggle with—your fears, insecurities, irritations, and worries. In this chapter, we will define what is in that left hand—the ways you most want to be in your relationships, work, and life in general. We will develop skills for keeping our focus on moving toward that left hand, rather than spending our time trying to figure out how to control and manage those difficult feelings in the right hand.

What Do We Mean by Values?

In ACT, values are defined as "freely chosen, verbally constructed consequences of ongoing, dynamic, evolving, patterns of activity" (Dahl 2015). Put more plainly, we can think of values as how you want to be in areas of your life that have meaning for you. Most of the time, our values are unique to us, even if our family, culture, geographical location, or other forces influenced our caring about them. Values can help guide our behavior, and by using the exercises in this chapter, we can bring the power of values to our choices every day.

A fun way to start the process of exploring your personal values is this modification of an exercise developed by Laura King in a research study called the Best Possible Future Self exercise (2001).

EXERCISE: Best Possible Future Self

Imagine it is some point in the future, and all your hopes, dreams, goals, and aspirations have come true. In the space below, describe what your life would look like: Where would you be? What would you be doing with your day? Who would be in your life? What would you do in your spare time? What else do you notice? Try to include as much detail as possible, not just about the fun stuff (what kind of car you drive), but also really spend time thinking about *how you are* (generous, caring, adventurous, loyal) in your relationships, in your job, and in your activities. Remember, there's no reality here, just describe what your best possible future would look like.

When I picture the future if everything worked out the best way it could, I imagine…

_____

_____

_____

_____

_____

_____

_____

_____

This exercise paints a broad picture of what an optimal life looks like for you. Take a minute to focus on the parts of the exercise that say something about what is most important to you. Circle any words in your writing that describe how you want to *be* (generous, loving, hard-working, creative, active, fun). We'll use them below to help further define what matters the most to you.

Defining Your Personal Values

Now that we know some things about what you most want your life to be like in the future, we can start to see what actual values are most important to you. Look at the words you circled, what do you notice? Are there themes? It is important to see where your values come up the most, and which domains of your life contain specific values, like relationships or your career.

To define your values in these domains, we can use a classic ACT exercise to explore specific values in the various aspects of your life: romantic relationships, family relationships, friendships, work, education, fun, spirituality, contributing to society, and physical well-being. The goal for this exercise is to describe the "you" that you most want to be—not necessarily the "you" you are now. Also, these values should be adjectives and general directions, rather than specific actions. For example, a value might be a general aspiration, like being a loving parent, rather than a specific action, like giving your child a hug.

EXERCISE: How Do You Want to Be?

For each prompt, write a few words that describe what you *aspire* to be in your life in relation to that area. Again, think of adjectives for how you want to be (loving, adventurous, consistent) rather than specific things or experiences you want to have. If you aren't connected to a particular area, you can skip it, although if it's an area you'd like to have as a bigger part of your life later on, it is great to include your values even if it isn't something you have been living (e.g., if you are without a partner right now, but would like to be a partner who is loving, caring, and affectionate in the future).

Here are some example words to get you started (but remember to really think about what is most important to you): loving, generous, thoughtful, kind, light-hearted, connected, reliable, adventurous, consistent, helpful, conscientious, curious, present, active, dependable, fun, spontaneous, honest, intentional, caring, open, trusting, giving, compassionate, supportive, loyal, or playful.

In the area of romantic relationships, I aspire to be a partner who is:

_____

_____

_____

In the area of friendships, I aspire to be a friend who is:

_____

_____

_____

In the area of family relationships, I aspire to be a family member who is:

_____

_____

_____

In the area of work, I aspire to be an employee who is:

_____

_____

_____

In the area of education and learning, I aspire to be someone who is:

_____

_____

_____

In the area of fun and recreation, I aspire to be someone who is:

_____

_____

_____

In the area of spirituality, religion, and faith, I aspire to be someone who is:

_____

_____

_____

In the area of how I take care of myself physically, I aspire to be someone who is:

_____

_____

_____

In the area of volunteering, contributing, or giving back, I aspire to be someone who is:

_____

_____

_____

What did you notice? What themes were present in what you wrote? Were there some values you feel you are already living out? Any values or themes that you noticed you want to bring more focus to?

_____

_____

_____

_____

_____

This exercise can give you a lot more information about how you want to be in your life, but it can be a little overwhelming to think about how to implement all those values at the same time. So, before we get to that, let's explore a way to quickly access your values right now—or any time you want to keep your values close at hand.

EXERCISE: Give Me Five

How do you want to be right now? Like, literally today? If you could jump forward in time to a week from now, what would you most want to look back and see about how you were *today*?

Let's look at the day you're in right now. Maybe it's a weekend and you have the rest of the day to take care of anything that comes up. Maybe it's a weekday and you're hard at work. Maybe you're in therapy right now and planning what comes next. What are the most important values you hold for yourself today? List five adjectives *you would want to describe you* for the rest of the day today. Starting now. Try to count them off on your fingers and remember them. Then, at the end of the day, check in to see how you did.

Remember, only one (adjective) word on each line!

(Jen's Example) Today I aspire to be:	Today I aspire to be:
1. Present	1. _____
2. Active	2. _____
3. Loving	3. _____
4. Understanding	4. _____
5. Focused	5. _____

What did you notice? Do you see an overlap with the more comprehensive values assessment you did above? Sometimes key values show up over and over, and sometimes what is most important to us is more based on circumstances and what we're doing. Keeping this short "five fingers" list of values in mind is a good way to bring your values with you throughout the day.

Differentiating Values, Goals, and Actions

In our normal use of language, the concepts of "values" and "goals" have a lot of overlap. If I ask you about your romantic relationship values, you may answer by saying that you want to get married or have a long-term relationship. From an ACT perspective, these answers refer to goals, not values, because they can be completed. Goals are defined as concrete consequences of our actions that can be obtained or finished, whereas values are directions we can head in, but never reach.

With this in mind, if I asked you again about your romantic relationship values, you might say, "being a loving partner" or "being considerate and understanding with my partner." If you value "being loving," you might work on goals that will move you toward that value (joining a dating app if you are single, spending meaningful time with a partner, showing your partner how much you care for them). Your value of being loving doesn't change and you don't ever "achieve" it, you are just moving in the direction of it.

Goals help us move toward our values, but they aren't a replacement for them. Take again the example of valuing being loving. If you begin seeking a relationship without bringing in the value behind it, you run the risk of having your dates be more motivated by an attempt to control your negative feelings (loneliness, feeling left out when other people are in relationships, insecurity). In other words, dating becomes part of the cycle of control we talked about in chapter 1. Rather than bringing the vitality that comes from moving toward your values, dating becomes more constricting and more life-shrinking.

EXERCISE: Goal Up

Goals are most effective when they are paired with personal values (Chase et al. 2013). Take your most important values from the exercises above and generate related goals. Remember, values are general directions (being a thoughtful friend) and goals are specific destinations in the direction of the value (calling to check in on a friend who is struggling).

Most important values:	Related goals:

And... Action!

While it can be problematic to focus exclusively on goals to move our behavior, all is not lost for the goal-oriented person. When we define our most important values, we also can think about the steps we want to take to move toward those values. For example, if I aspire to be an active person (value) and want to start exercising more (goal), I can create lots of action steps to move me toward my value little by little. I can join a gym (action), sign up for an exercise class (action), stop by after work to lift weights (action), run for fifteen minutes on the treadmill (action)—you get the idea.

EXERCISE: Values, Goals, Actions

Another classic values tool used in ACT is the assessment of specific goals and actions for each value. This exercise will help you define specific steps to take to live out each of your important values. This is particularly important for generating committed action steps and increasing overall vitality.

Given the values you established above, generate some goals for each value, and then some specific actions you can take to live your values in an ongoing way. Remember that values should be general directions, goals should be destinations along the way, and actions should be concrete, specific things you could do today.

Value	Goals	Actions
Example: Being a loving partner	Be more expressive of warm feelings	Calling during the day to say "I love you," spontaneous hugs, expressing appreciation

This exercise sometimes causes people to feel pressured to do more toward their values or feel like the actions they could take toward their values are too small or insignificant. If you notice those reactions, just keep moving forward. Remember that these are directions we are continuously heading toward, and the *journey itself* is where our vitality comes from.

Core Relationship Values

Relationships are crucial to human beings, but they also are an area where we can have strong "negative" feelings, like disappointment, shame, grief, and fear of rejection. We often act in ways that are not consistent with our values in order to "manage" our relationships or the feelings that come with them.

EXERCISE: Adjectives Exercise—Relationships

Think about all the different types of relationships you have—partner, ex-partner, friend, grandchild, son, daughter, child, sister, brother, sibling, cousin, niece, nephew, mother, father, parent, guardian, aunt, uncle, grandparent, coworker, neighbor. Maybe you are a fellow parishioner, a student, a volunteer, a teammate, or a club member.

These relationships might all be different, and you may have different values that you want to live out in each of them, but often there are uniting core ideals we have for ourselves across all our relationships. In the spaces below, list some of your most important values. Remember to stay focused at the values (adjectives) level, and to keep your focus on your own role, rather than the other person's.

In my romantic relationships, I aspire to be:	In my friendships, I aspire to be:
1. _____	1. _____
2. _____	2. _____
3. _____	3. _____
4. _____	4. _____
5. _____	5. _____

In my family relationships I aspire to be:	As a _____, I aspire to be:
1. _____	1. _____
2. _____	2. _____
3. _____	3. _____
4. _____	4. _____
5. _____	5. _____

Do you notice any patterns? What are the most important values you hold across all your relationships?

_____

Staying in Your Own Lane in Relationships

Another challenge in important relationships is our tendency to sometimes want to change the behavior (and feelings) of the other person. Our ability to live our values can feel tied to what the other person does. For example, in therapy, we often hear things like "I can't be a loving partner because my spouse doesn't do enough to help out" or "Even though I value being present and focused at work, my partner will think I don't care if I don't respond to their texts right away, so I end up spending lots of time texting them back while I'm at work."

Many of us are taught from an early age to assume responsibility for other people's feelings and to tie our behavior to what is happening for people around us. This, however, often gets in the way of living our personal values. One way to combat this is to intentionally tie our behavior to our values, and recognize that the other person's experience is not on our side of the street. In other words, instead of checking whether our behavior made the other person happy, we can ask ourselves: "Did I show up in a way I value with that person today, whether it changed anything or not? Did I keep my focus on my side of the street?"

EXERCISE: What Do You Want Your Side of the Street to Look Like?

Think about situations where you struggle with someone in your life. Write down your situation in the first column, then see if you can identify some of your key values for the relationship in the first gray column, and then describe their side of the street (the parts you have no business trying to control) in the second gray column. Finally, write about how you might live your values in this situation in the last column.

Situation/conflict	My side	Other person's side	How I can live my values
My partner is impatient with how slowly I respond to texts when I'm at work	I value being productive and focused at work, and also value being a responsive and present partner	My partner's impatience	Kindly let my partner know that I won't respond during work, and create a plan in case of emergency. Let go of anything beyond that

This exercise lets us define where our values are—and where they are not—in tricky situations with others. Thinking about these situations ahead of time prevents us from responding reactively or giving in to other person's requests in a way that isn't consistent with our values.

Defining Willingness Targets for Your Values

When you begin defining your values, you may notice that there are areas where a strong value and a lot of difficult emotions seem to go hand in hand. For example, if you aspire to be an open, nonjudgmental parent, you may struggle with anxiety and fear about what will happen to your child if you don't provide a lot of feedback and guidance.

Recently, researchers have begun to investigate the relationship between difficult emotions and values more carefully. One interesting study explored whether values are related to our willingness to experience pain (Páez-Blarrina et al. 2008). Two groups of participants received a painful shock (but not one that could harm them). The first group was asked to think about a time in their life when they did something painful because it was important to them. The second group thought about a time that they quit something because it was painful. Both groups reported equal amounts of pain from the shock, but the individuals who were directed to think of a time when pain and values were related chose to receive more and greater shocks. Additionally, the participants elected to continue receiving shocks despite experiencing "very much pain," indicating that the shocks were still painful, but participants no longer believed that they needed to stop them.

This study highlights the connection between values and pain. If you're going to live a life according to your values, pain will inevitably come along. There's no way to avoid it. Pulling away from pain tends to pull us away from values as well. Steve Hayes, the cofounder of ACT, says, "You hurt where you care and you care where you hurt." We think that sums it up quite nicely.

EXERCISE: You Hurt Where You Care and You Care Where You Hurt

Do a little exploring of some areas in your life that are very important to you and the pain—big or small—that comes along as you engage them.

We will show you some examples from our lives:

Matt

Area of life	What you find meaningful	What's hard
My relationship with my wife	Having someone who really knows me and has my back in all things. Plus, she's hella funny.	When she is sad or anxious, I feel uncomfortable. I want to make it better, but I know that all I can do is be loving. But it's hard to see someone I love suffer.
My work as a therapist	I get to get to know people deeply and help them through hard times.	I hear some pretty difficult stuff, and sometimes it's hard to let it go. Though I love helping people change and grow, it sometimes hurts my heart to know some of the difficult things they have gone through.
My life as a musician and creative person	When I was seven or eight years old, I wanted more than anything else to be a rock star. I don't care about being a rock star now, but I love to make music, play guitar, sing, and write songs.	For every day I'm totally thrilled with my capacity to make music, there is also a day when I feel frustrated by what I can't do. I also have to limit myself because of chronic pain in my hands.

Jen

Area of life	What you find meaningful	What's hard
My role as a mom	The love and incredible connection I feel with my kids.	When they struggle or are vulnerable or in danger, I feel scared and overwhelmed by the desire to take away their suffering and keep them safe.
My spiritual practice	My practice has helped me stay present and intentional through the many difficult things that have come along in my life.	I experience bouts of doubt, agitation, low motivation, and self-criticism when I practice.
My work as a therapist for people at the end of life	I am honored to get to help people during such an important time in their lives.	I experience grief and pain from the loss of so many people I care deeply about.

Now it's your turn:

Area of life	What you find meaningful	What's hard

Area of life	What you find meaningful	What's hard

What do you notice about what you wrote?

_____

_____

_____

_____

_____

_____

Commitment

When we talk about values in ACT, we typically focus on two main skills: clarifying personal values and taking committed action toward those values. While some people just require the defining and clarifying of values and they are on their way, most of us need some specific exercises to help bring those values into our daily lives.

EXERCISE: How Small Can You Get?

Think about an important value that you want to prioritize working on in your life. Maybe this is a value you haven't thought much about or one that you do pretty well on already, but it is important enough that you want to maintain a high level of priority for it. Use the space below to define the smallest step you could take today toward that value. Follow that with the next smallest step toward that value, and so on.

Let's say, for example, you want to work on your value of being a more spiritually connected. The smallest step to take today might be to pray or meditate for a few minutes. The smallest step tomorrow might be to pray or meditate for fifteen minutes. The smallest step the day after tomorrow might be to pray or meditate for twenty minutes. The following day it might to pray or meditate for twenty minutes and find a church or meditation center to check out.

	Done?
Target Value:	
Smallest step today:	
Smallest step tomorrow:	
Smallest step the next day:	
Smallest step the next day:	
Smallest step the next day:	
Smallest step the next day:	

What did you notice? Maybe you noticed that imagining taking small steps does not always feel as good as imagining accomplishing big ones. We like to set high goals for ourselves, even when they aren't possible. In the space below, reflect on your reaction to taking small steps, and write about how you can use your small steps in your own values to build momentum.

_____

_____

_____

_____

_____

_____

_____

_____

_____

_____

_____

_____

Differentiating Between Process and Outcome

Just as we talked about how goals are sometimes used to control our unwanted thoughts and feelings, we can also utilize our values in a way that makes them less useful. For example, we can become very focused on the idea of being a good partner *so our partner appreciates us*, or being a good parent *so our children will behave better*. These actions, then, become less about our values and more about—you guessed it—control.

One way we can think about this is values are about the *process* of living them to grow and enhance meaningful living, not about the *outcomes* that may occur as you do so. Sadly, we can't control outcomes.

Let's take an example. Let's say you value being a thoughtful partner, and the word "thoughtful" came up right away when you were defining your values above. And let's say that after doing the exercises in this book, you decide to engage in some thoughtful behaviors with your partner—you make their favorite meal, you wash their socks, and you encourage them before their big meeting. If you are engaging in those values-driven actions at a process level, then you are doing them for the purpose of living your values. Thus, you are checking your behavior against your values and finding that there is a match, which feels good and will increase the future probability that you will engage in the same behaviors in the future. This should lead to an upward spiral of value-driven behaviors and good-for-me feelings.

But if you are engaging in those same values-driven actions at an outcome level, then you are doing them for the purpose of producing a different outcome. Now you are checking your behaviors against how well they worked—did they make your partner happy? Was your partner appreciative? Did that make you happy? The problem with this is obvious: you have no control over whether your behaviors make your partner happy or appreciative. Therefore, your actions only "work" if a specific response is delivered by the other person, and they can die out if your partner doesn't comment or says something snarky. No upward spiral.

EXERCISE: Process Versus Outcome

Look at some of the values, goals, and actions you defined in the exercise above. Write down how you can help yourself stay focused on the process of these goals, rather than the outcome.

For example, if you have a *value* of being a supportive friend, and a *goal* of being a better communicator, you might well have generated an *action* of calling to check in with them periodically. However, with this action, you might need to watch out for becoming too focused on whether the phone call goes well or whether they call you back or appreciate the call. Instead, you will want to check in with yourself about *why* you are remembering to call your friends to check in with them—that way, you can make sure that you are living your supportive friend value.

Value: _____ Goal: _____ Action: _____

"Outcome focus" to watch out for:

_____

_____

_____

"Process focus" to remember and check in with myself about:

_____

_____

_____

Value: _____ Goal: _____ Action: _____

"Outcome focus" to watch out for:

_____

_____

_____

"Process focus" to remember and check in with myself about:

_____

_____

_____

Value: _____ Goal: _____ Action: _____

"Outcome focus" to watch out for:

_____

_____

_____

"Process focus" to remember and check in with myself about:

_____

_____

_____

It is important to remember that sometimes, focusing on the outcome of an action makes sense. For example, if you are playing basketball, the important part is getting the ball in the hoop and scoring, not whether you had a good process in throwing the ball. In the same way, there are times when focusing on outcomes will move you toward your values. Generally, though, focusing on process will give you a piece you can do something about, even when the seas of life are rough.

EXERCISE: Choose, Choose, and Choose Again

One thing we know for sure is that it is hard to do anything with consistency—life is always getting in the way. Use the space below to write a note to yourself, reminding yourself why you choose to move in the direction of your values, even when things get difficult.

Dear me,

Here is why moving toward my values matters to me, even when I don't feel like it.

_____

_____

_____

_____

_____

_____

_____

_____

_____

_____

_____

_____

Summing It Up

Clarifying personal values and taking intentional, committed actions to move toward them is the cornerstone of the work we do in ACT. All the other processes and interventions in ACT are designed to support movement toward a more values-driven and meaningful life. Coming in to the present, defusing from our thoughts, practicing willingness toward difficult experiences, and developing more flexible perspective taking all allow us to purposefully move in the direction of our values. In this chapter we defined what those values are and ways to take intentional steps toward them, so that the vitality of living authentically can take over.

CHAPTER 6

Flexible Perspective-Taking Skills

You Are More Than You Think You Are

If you were given an assignment to answer the question "Who am I?" how would you answer? This is a really big question. You might define yourself by your roles: mother, father, auntie, brother, child, coach, friend, boss, assistant branch manager, teammate, etc. Or you might define yourself by your vocation(s): barista, furniture maker, mechanic, lawyer, firefighter, dog walker, accountant, hospice worker, and so on. You might also offer some narratives that describe who you are: "I'm a good person," "I'm a loving mother," "I'm a hard worker," "I'm an anxious person," "I'm no good at commitment," "My hardships have made me who I am," and on and on. Where would you end? Is there a definitive collection of roles, behaviors, experiences, and stories that make up the real you? Where does your "self" begin and end?

Many academic and pop psychology theories offer some kind of way to find your true self. But ACT doesn't. ACT kind of sidesteps the issue, leaving it to the philosophers. The emphasis is instead on encouraging you to build skills that undermine the many ways we can get stuck in narrow ideas of who we are, which also means approaching the idea of "self" a bit more flexibly than we're often taught. ACT does this to free you, so you are less driven by passing thoughts and feelings, and more capable of taking action devoted to your values.

For example, have you ever met someone who has a narrative about themselves that keeps them in a box? A narrative like "I have low self-esteem," "I'm no good at commitment," "I have impostor syndrome," "I can't do that—it's just too hard." These narratives, though completely normal and inevitable (see chapter 2 on defusion), can become self-fulfilling prophecies that limit the possibilities for our lives.

Instead of trying to find a better narrative about the self, or some kind of true self, ACT offers a set of skills that help us do the following:

- Let go of over-identifying with painful thoughts and feelings—for example, feeling like our anxiety, anger, or inner self-critic define us

- Reduce our tendency to be limited by stories about who we are and what we're capable of

- Expand the possibilities of who we can choose to be, moment to moment, in our *actions* and *intentions*, no matter what shows up inside of us

This set of skills is called "flexible perspective taking," and it starts with learning to take the "observer" perspective, also known as the "observing self," which we will get to next. You don't have to understand why it's a "self" just yet. Just focus on learning to take this perspective. We will try it out in a couple of ways. Here's the first one.

You Are Distinct from Your Thoughts and Feelings

Think of a time in your life where you had a noticeable emotional reaction—something recent. If you're feeling something right now, that's even better. Have you got it? Now, write the situation that triggered this reaction on the line below.

We are now going to break your emotional reaction down into its components: feelings and sensations, urges and actions, and thoughts and images. If you need extra guidance, there are a couple of examples provided.

Situation: _____

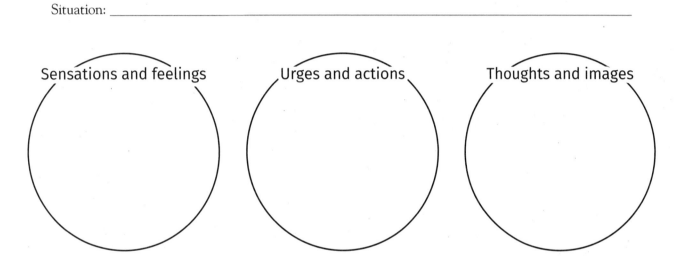

Sensations and feelings   Urges and actions   Thoughts and images

Sensations and feelings. In the lefthand circle, write down all the feelings and sensations that you experienced with this emotional reaction. By feelings and sensations, we mean the stuff that shows up in your body, like tension in your neck, a pit in your stomach, a heaviness in your chest, that feeling you get around your eyes when you're about to cry, or that buzzing sensation you get throughout your body when you're nervous. Take your time and record anything you think you might have experienced in this area.

Urges and actions. Next, move on to urges and actions. Actions are the things you do that are observable to other people, and urges are the embodied feelings that go along with your actions, whether or not you actually do the action. So, for example, you might have the urge to respond defensively to a terse, critical text from your boss, but you might not actually do so, knowing it's probably best to take a deep breath before crafting a response. Urges might include the desire to run away, the desire to say something mean, or the desire to curl up in a ball. Actions might be big, like actually running away, or small, like slumping your shoulders, tapping your feet, or frowning.

Thoughts and images. Finally, write down all the thoughts and images that were going through your mind at that time. It sometimes helps to make thoughts into sentences even though our minds don't always work that way. The thought could be something like "This always happens to me" or "Why is he so annoying?" or "What's gonna happen if I fail?" Thoughts can also be images and memories. So, you might write something like "The image of me failing my test."

Now here's the fun part. Take a look at your sensations and feelings, urges and actions, and thoughts and images on this page. Imagine that you could actually take these experiences out of yourself and place them in front of you like we have modeled here.

And now, without thinking too hard about it, notice the difference between you, the one who is looking at these thoughts, feelings, and actions, and the thoughts, feelings, and actions themselves. There's *you*, and then there are your internal experiences and external actions. Notice that distinction and sit with it for a few moments.

The Difference Between You and What You Experience

Okay, we understand if you're thinking this is kind of silly. Of course you are not the same thing as what's written on the page. But if you can see the distinction between those marks on the page and you, the human being looking at them, you can start to build the ability to see a similar distinction between your actual thoughts, feelings, sensations, and urges, and *you*, the whole human being who experiences them. This is the observer perspective: looking at your momentary thoughts, feelings, and behaviors as if they are distinct from you, the whole, continuous, stable person who experiences them.

Have you ever heard the saying, "You are not your thoughts and feelings"? This is what it means. It's not a philosophical claim. It's a perspective. It's actually more ACT-like to say you are *much more* than your thoughts and feelings.

EXAMPLES

Here are some examples of emotional reactions, both pleasant and painful, broken down into their components.

Situation: Meeting my kittens Georgia and Finley at the front door when I get home each day

Sensations and feelings

face flushed,

excited,

that "squee" feeling when you see something cute

Urges and actions

crouched down,

smiled,

opened eyes wide,

shouted "Hello Georgia! Hello Finley!"

Thoughts and images

"Oh my God, they are so cute!" "They're getting so big!" Images of them just a few weeks ago.

Situation: Boss tells me they are unhappy with my performance

Sensations and feelings

face flushed,

sinking feeling in my stomach,

tension in my arms and shoulders

Urges and actions

Sat silently, nodding and listening,

urge to defend myself,

urge to make a joke to lighten things

Thoughts and images

Racing thoughts, "I've been working really hard – this is BS!" "He doesn't see my real value."

The Place You Watch Your Thoughts and Feelings From

Now let's try this again with whatever's going on for you right now, in this moment. You don't have to write anything down in circles. Just follow the steps and name the experiences to yourself. And as you do so, look at these experiences in your mind's eye just as you might look at the circles. It helps if you do this kind of slowly; that way, you don't miss what's going on.

Notice what sensations and feelings you are experiencing right now. Name them silently to yourself. Close your eyes if you need to and give it a few moments before you go on to the next prompt.

Now notice the part of you that is watching these sensations and feelings from the inside. There's a place from which we "look" at what we are experiencing inside, a place where our consciousness seems to be. Sometimes it's referred to as your "mind's eye." For most of us, it's behind our eyes somewhere. Tune into that place. Notice it for a few moments, and notice that it is different from the sensations and feelings that you were watching.

And now, with eyes open or closed, notice what urges and actions you are experiencing right now. Name them silently to yourself. Give it a few moments before you go on to the next prompt.

Now, again, notice the place inside you from which you are watching these urges and actions. Tune into that place. Notice it for a few moments, and notice that it is different from the urges and behaviors that you were watching.

Finally, with eyes open or closed, notice what thoughts and images are going through your head right now. Name them silently to yourself. Give it a few moments before you go on to the next prompt.

And again, notice the place inside you from which you are watching these thoughts and images. Tune into that place. Notice it for a few moments, and notice that it is different from the thoughts and images that you are watching.

If you get stuck, go back to looking at objects in your environment, and notice the place inside you, usually behind your eyes, where you are registering those objects. Then go back to doing the same thing with your internal experiences—thoughts, feelings, urges, etc.

When you not only notice what you are experiencing but also recognize the place from which you are "looking" at your experiences, that's also taking the observer's perspective.

Do some reflecting on what you noticed.

_____

_____

_____

_____

_____

_____

_____

_____

What All This Has to Do with the "Self"

So far, we've shown you the observer's perspective in two different ways. The first is that that there's *you*, and then there's *what you experience inside*, and these are different from one another. The second is that there is a place from which you can look out at all of your experiences, kind of like the cockpit of an airplane or the bridge of the starship Enterprise. But remember, we started this chapter by saying that ACT has a unique way of helping you sidestep narrow conceptions of "Who I am." So, what do these perspectives have to do with the "self?"

Well, as we noted earlier, another name for this observer's perspective is the "observing self." It's not your real self or true self. It's simply a metaphorical part of you that you can access to get some distance from painful thoughts and feelings when things get rough. It's also a part of you that is different from your roles, your vocations, and all the stories you have about yourself. It's the place from which you notice all of those other parts of you. As we noted earlier, we humans can get overidentified with these parts of ourselves, believing deeply in self-limiting stories like "I'm a victim of trauma," or viewing our depression or anxiety as *who we are*. The observer's perspective is the first place we can step back to notice that we are more than those stories.

There will be more to say about this further in this chapter. In the meantime, if you want to go a bit deeper into the observing self experientially, try out the "observing self" meditation in the online resources. However, if you've never done any mindfulness meditation before, you might want to start with reading chapter 3 on present moment awareness and trying out the simpler exercises like "Introduction to Mindfulness."

From Observer to Container

As you start taking the observer's perspective—or in other words, connecting with your observing self—you'll notice that it sometimes seems not just as if you are distinct from thoughts and feelings, but also kind of like you are a container of sorts, and your thoughts and feelings are just stuff inside you. Let's illustrate this with a few metaphors popular in the ACT world:

Vase metaphor. You are like a big, sturdy vase. Your thoughts and feelings are the flowers inside. The vase has been around for a long time, changing very little. But many, many flowers have inhabited that vase. All of them have come and gone throughout the life of the vase. The flowers are not the vase, they are simply inhabitants, and temporary ones at that.

House metaphor. You are like an old, sturdy house. Your thoughts and feelings are the inhabitants, furnishings, and decor. The house has been around for a long time, staying pretty much the same. But throughout the years, different inhabitants have come and gone, the furnishings have changed, and the decor has evolved. The house is always the house, no matter what is going on inside of it.

Sky metaphor. You are like the sky. Thoughts and feelings are like the weather. Clouds, rain, thunderstorms, lightning, tornadoes, and even sunlight and moonlight are always changing. But the sky is always there. The sky is never harmed by the weather. No matter what is going on in the sky—no matter how tumultuous the weather—somewhere up above, there is still blue sky.

There are lots of similar metaphors inside ACT and other mindfulness-based treatments, like the mountain metaphor—and this is also the case in the spiritual traditions from which these treatments draw many of their techniques. Search the words "mountain" and "sky" in your favorite meditation app, and you'll find a bunch of results.

The following exercise is a useful strategy to cultivate this sense of being the container of all you experience, while taking action in the service of what's important to you.

EXERCISE: Mapping Your Thoughts and Feelings

This exercise can be quite useful for when want help approaching something difficult you might be avoiding or dealing with a situation that that regularly makes you miserable. I (Matt) work primarily with students at a medical university. Many of my students show up in my office stressed out about some task that they are procrastinating on—studying for an exam, getting started on a project, or emailing an intimidating professor. We could talk all day about how they just need to get started—they know that! But that's not the same as getting started. So instead, we actually *get started*, in real time, combining all the facets of the observer's perspectives along the way.

You can do this too, and it can relate to anything in your life, big or small: calling your extra-critical family member to say hi, looking at your credit score, sending an email apologizing for something, standing up for yourself—anything that makes your stomach squeeze a little bit.

Materials needed:

- Stack of sticky notes

- Magic marker or similarly thick pen

- Large, open surface like a tabletop, a stretch of floor, or a bare wall on which to put your sticky notes

This exercise involves labeling all the thoughts and feelings that come up around the difficult situation one at a time on individual sticky notes and laying them out in front of you so that you can see them from a birds-eye view. Then, if there's a meaningful action to take, you can take that action surrounded by all of your thoughts and feelings without giving them any extra energy.

If you are like one of the students I work with who procrastinates, it might look a little bit like what's on the next page. Notice all the self-criticisms, uncomfortable feelings, and dire images. When I conduct this exercise, once my client has mapped all of that stuff out on sticky notes—usually on their laptop or the desk where they work—they practice initiating a project without the typical dwelling, spiraling, or avoiding that usually happens. I think it helps that I'm there with them the first time, so you might want to consider doing this with a friend nearby.

Center yourself. Start by taking a few deep breaths and letting them out slowly to center yourself in this moment. This exercise will bring you a little bit closer to some painful thoughts and feelings. But remember: you are not your thoughts and feelings; you are *much more* than your thoughts and feelings.

Contact the hard situation. Now, imagine a situation in your life that's difficult for you, one you're willing to do some work with right now. See if you can make it real—put yourself right in the middle of the situation, experiencing the sights, sounds, thoughts, feelings, and sensations you usually encounter or will likely encounter when it occurs. And if you are actually in the middle of the situation is it's happening in real time—for example, if you're about to make a difficult phone call, get started on something you're avoiding, or ask your boss for a raise—you likely have access to all of those thoughts and feelings without even trying.

Label your thoughts and feelings on your sticky notes. Next, one at a time, and at a slowish pace, start labeling each internal experience (thought, image, feeling, sensation, memory, urge) that you notice on a separate sticky note, placing them in front of you on whatever surface you've chosen.

As you do the exercise, notice a few things:

- You are not your thoughts and feelings—they are simply part of you.

- These experiences, though seemingly powerful, are habitual and will eventually pass.

- You are bigger than these experiences—literally. There's you, then there are these sticky notes, which are much smaller than you.

- These experiences don't have to dictate your actions. You can have them and take action at the same time.

Take the next step(s). Finally, if you are using this exercise to help yourself get started on something you've been avoiding, take the first step. You can set a timer for a minute and spend that minute opening your email, finding the phone number you need to call, opening up a web browser, writing a list of things you want to say—whatever it is you need to do.

After a minute, see if there any other sticky notes you can create. Did anything else show up for you? Feel free to label those things as well.

Do this a few more times—as many times as needed—and when it feels right, just continue doing the task without stopping anymore.

When the task is done, do some reflecting. What did you notice?

With my students, I encourage them to keep their sticky notes around as a sign that they can have these thoughts and feelings *and*:

- Do the next important thing

- Take action that is different from where their thoughts and feelings are leading them

- Do something that follows from their values

They don't have to wait around for these thoughts and feelings to go away before they can get moving.

"I've waited way too long to get to this."	Urge to go do something else—check social media, get another cup of coffee, etc.	Heaviness in my chest
Comparing myself to other people who "have their act together"	"I'm never going to finish this project."	"Why am I so lazy?"
The image of a great big red "F" written on the front page	Shame	Anxiety
"Just quit whining and get started!"	The image of my family members looking disappointed	Mind racing

Disentangling from Self-Limiting "Who I Am" Stories

Now that you've had a lot of practice taking the observer's perspective, let's get more deeply into this "self" stuff we've been referring to throughout the chapter. We have been preparing with the observer perspective to help you notice where narratives about "who you are" might be getting in the way of living your most meaningful life.

EXERCISE: Naming Your Stories

We all have stories about who we are: "I'm a redhead," "I'm codependent," "I am a good person," "I'm much more intellectual than these people," "My religious upbringing made me who I am," "I've always been much more reserved than my sister." We could do this all day. Think about some of the stories you have. Using the prompts on the next page, see if you can fill as many blanks as you can after the prompts given—and whatever other prompts you can imagine. See if you can come up with as many as you can, even seemingly innocuous ones (e.g., "I am a lover of fancy, way-too-expensive coffee").

I... _____

I... _____

I... _____

I... _____

I... _____

I... _____

I... _____

I... _____

I... _____

I am... _____

I am... _____

I am... _____

I am... _____

I am... _____

I am... _____

I am... _____

I am... _____

I am... _____

I am a... _____

I am a... _____

I am a... _____

I am a... _____

I am a... _____

I am a... _____

I am a... _____

I am a... _____

I am a... _____

I always… _____

I always… _____

I always… _____

I always… _____

I always… _____

I always… _____

I always… _____

I always… _____

I never… _____

I never… _____

I never… _____

I never… _____

I never… _____

I never… _____

I never… _____

Other: _____

Other: _____

Other: _____

Once you have completed these sentences, look over the stories you wrote down, and look for the following:

Recurring themes. For example, you might notice that many of your stories (e.g., I'm no good at relationships, I am a middling father, I'm just good enough at my job) are connected to a core idea, such as you are defective in some way. (By the way, having a sense that you are defective in some way is *pretty darn common*, so if you look for it, you will probably see it.)

Roles or evaluations that feel essential to who you are. For example, I'm embarrassed to say that I (Matt) carry around the story "I am a smart person." I will lift heaven and earth to prove to you that I am smart. Sometimes it's useful; many times, people just wish I would keep my mouth closed, or I end up taking up a lot of space where other people could be talking or contributing.

EXERCISE: How Do These Stories Work for You?

Pick a few stories that seem to stick out as problematic, and answer the following questions.

How does each story prevent you from taking action according to your values? For example, a story like "I'm undesirable" might get in the way of dating.

How does each story narrow your life? For example, a story like "I'm a man, and I don't do feelings" might prevent you from really connecting with others.

_____

_____

_____

_____

_____

_____

_____

How would you be living differently *today* if each of these stories were no longer there?

_____

_____

_____

_____

_____

_____

_____

_____

Was there a time when these stories helped you in some way? Maybe they protected you, gave you a sense of identity, or something else.

_____

_____

_____

_____

_____

_____

_____

_____

Is there a place in your life where these stories might still be helpful, even if they don't work for you most of the time?

_____

_____

_____

_____

_____

_____

_____

Notice that at no time do we say that you need to change your story or find a new story. As usual, we are just looking at workability—how does it operate? Where does it work for you? Where does it fail to work for you? If this is sounding a lot like defusion (chapter 2), you're right. All we are doing here is defusing from stories about "who you are."

You will discover that as you live your life in a more values-driven way, you will become more and more the person you want to be. But you will always be "becoming"—you will never arrive.

True to Your Values, Not Your "Self"

So now, when you find yourself thinking things like, "I've got to be true to myself" or "That's just not me," or "I'm not that guy," see if you can shift those thoughts around into statements about values.

Some questions you could ask yourself in the moment, no matter who your mind says you are, could be: What would I be doing if I were living my values in this situation? How do I want to be? How do I want to show up? What actions would I be taking *right now*? This is about being *true to your values*—a way of thinking that we argue provides a much more flexible and adaptive way of responding to life. In a sense, we are saying, "Be the you that you *choose* to be—in your actions—not the you that your mind says you are."

By the way, you have a whole chapter on values right before this one (chapter 5) to go back to if you're struggling with how to find or live your values.

Taking the Perspective of Others

Whew! Now that we've determined that you are not necessarily who your mind thinks you are, and we have also practiced disidentifying with thoughts and feelings that sometimes feel like they are the sum of us, we finally have the room to start taking other perspectives. Here are some exercises we find especially useful for helping people break out of their ruts, broaden their range of behavior, and take new, values-driven actions.

EXERCISE: An Older, Wiser You

Sometimes when things are tough, it's hard to remember the big picture. Luckily, we can call on other versions of ourselves to help get perspective.

Think of a difficult place in your life right now: somewhere that you hurt a bit, feel confused, or tend to fall into old, unhelpful patterns of behavior. We are going to call on an older, wiser, more experienced version of you to help out. But first, write a little bit about the situation:

_____

_____

_____

_____

_____

_____

_____

_____

Now, imagine yourself twenty, thirty, or forty years in the future. This is a version of you that has grown wiser and more compassionate through experience, has lived a life closely connected to their values, and has let go of some of the internal struggles with thoughts and feelings that you still find yourself getting into.

Imagine what they look like. Imagine what they devote their energy to. And imagine what they would say to you about this situation if they could sit down with you over a cup of something warm in a cozy place and give you a big, squeezy hug.

Take a moment to write out their words: What would they encourage you to do? What would they encourage you to let go of? What words of encouragement might they offer? What words of validation might they offer? And what gestures of love might they offer you?

_____

_____

_____

_____

_____

_____

_____

_____

_____

_____

_____

This is an exercise you can do many times. Let this be a rough draft you come back to and revisit. See if you can really offer yourself what you need to hear, but in the kindest and most loving way.

EXERCISE: A Younger, Bolder You

For some people, another useful perspective is a younger, bolder, and less jaded version of themselves. Is there a version of you like this? I (Matt) think of my seven or eight-year-old self, who was always imagining an expansive world where anything could happen: he could be a rock star, a superhero, or the president of the United States. His feelings could be hurt pretty easily, but he also was pretty fearless, especially with people. He could make friends with anyone and loved new experiences.

As I've gotten older and dealt with hard things that life has offered, I've lost sight of some of that expansiveness. I've lost sight of some of that boldness. And I find it helpful to draw on that little guy, the one who was up for any adventure. I like to ask myself: What would he say? What would he do?

Do you have a version of yourself like this, or with some other lovely qualities that you could turn to again? If so, paint a vivid picture of that version of you.

_____

_____

_____

_____

_____

_____

_____

_____

Now think of something hard that you're going through, or someplace where you're stuck. Maybe it's a place where you're letting fear get in the way of living meaningfully. A place where life has gotten small instead of big. What might this younger, bolder version of you say to you? What gestures of love might they offer?

_____

_____

_____

_____

_____

_____

_____

_____

Again, let this be a rough draft you can come back to again and again. And try out hearing from yourself at other ages as well.

Endless Perspectives

There's no end to the perspectives you could take—both your own and those of other people. If you like, you can do the previous two exercises with any one of the perspectives below, all of which focus on the perspectives of other people.

- A compassionate mentor

- Someone who loves you very deeply

- Someone who has your best interests at heart, but doesn't agree with you

- Your beloved pet

- An older, wiser relative or friend, even if they have passed on

- A hero in your life—whether local (e.g., your high school football coach) or well-known (e.g., the Dalai Lama)

- The list is endless…

Summing It Up

There's quite a bit going on in this chapter, so let's walk you through it one last time.

The observing self/observer's perspective. It can help to practice flexible perspective taking by first learning the observer's perspective, also called the "observing self" or the "observer," which is a part of you that is *distinct from* what you think and feel.

The container perspective. Another perspective that follows closely from the observer perspective is the container perspective, in which we are the *whole*, and the thoughts, feelings, and sensations we experience are parts of the whole. Another way to say it is that you are *more than* what you think and feel.

Defusing from self-stories. If you can take these two perspectives, then it can become a whole lot easier to defuse (see chapter 2) from stories, narratives, and labels about who you are. Stories about the "self" can feel especially true. And therefore, they can be especially confining.

Who is the real me? Therefore, ACT sidesteps the question of "Who am I?" and asks different kinds of questions, such as, "Who do I want to be in this moment?" "How do I want to live my values?" and "How can I be true to my values?"

Switching perspectives. Taking the observer's perspective and holding our sense of "self" more lightly can open up room for taking other useful perspectives. That can mean the perspective of a version of us from many years from now, a version of us from many years ago, someone who loves us deeply, someone who is wise and compassionate, someone who challenges us, someone who knows us better than we know ourselves sometimes, our beloved furry friends, and on and on and on.

All of these perspectives work in tandem with other skills you've learned in this book to expand the possibilities for how you respond to your thoughts and feelings, as well as for how you act—both when things are hard in your life and when things are amazing. It's to the amazing that we turn next.

CHAPTER 7

Positive Psychology

Cultivating Values Related to Meaning, Pleasure, and Awe

Throughout this book, we provide skills for living our personal values while making room for difficult, scary, and painful experiences. In this chapter, we will focus instead on cultivating awareness and values related to amazing experiences—the values connected to broadening your experiences and enriching your life. We will draw on concepts of positive psychology, a subfield of psychological science focused on happiness, pleasure, and how human beings thrive and flourish (Seligman 2011).

Although they have similar end goals, ACT and positive psychology have slightly different ways of going about these goals. Positive psychology, in general, is focused on having more positive thoughts and feelings. More happiness, higher self-esteem, more peacefulness, and so on. In ACT, the goal is not having more positive experiences, but rather noticing all experiences and living in meaningful ways. So, not more "happiness" (an emotion) or "high self-esteem" (thoughts about self), or "peacefulness" (feeling or body sensation), but noticing those experiences when they are present (just as we notice the tough ones) and focusing on living out personal values.

If *reaching* for increased happiness worked as a general strategy, we would be all for it. Unfortunately, the reality is that focusing on "being happy" is often a self-defeating proposition. This is because being happy all the time is not possible. So, when happiness is the goal, we're a little more disappointed during the times when we're *not* feeling happy. Researchers have shown this in multiple ways. Mauss and colleagues (2011; 2012) have demonstrated that people who focused on happiness the most were less happy, and a little lonelier, than people who focused on happiness to a lesser degree.

Savoring

In chapter 3, we talked above the benefits of coming into the present moment to respond flexibly to difficult thoughts and feelings. The skill of coming into the present with awareness can be applied in many ways, and one of those ways is the idea of "savoring."

Savoring is anything we do that increases the intensity, duration, or overall appreciation of something we experience as positive. It can be thought of as the opposite of avoidance, but it's also the opposite of dampening down an experience, as we sometimes do with what's difficult. It is associated with higher levels of awareness in the best possible way. Try this little "taste" of it and see what we mean.

EXERCISE: Slow It Down

In this exercise, we will practice the task of savoring through the use of what is called "sensory-perceptual sharpening"—intentionally intensifying an experience by focusing on it. To do this, first track down something you want to eat or drink—it really doesn't matter what it is. It can be a cookie, a sandwich, a cup of tea—anything that you like.

First, look at the item. What color is it? What is its texture? What do you notice about it visually? What do you think it will taste like? Are you at all excited to try it? What does it feel like in your hand? What are the sensations in your fingers or hand as you hold it?

Now smell the object. What does it smell like? Is the smell strong or faint, or is there no smell at all? What does the air around it feel like when you breathe it in?

Next, taste it with the tip of your tongue. What does it feel like? Close your eyes and really pay attention to the sensations and experiences.

Now take a bite or drink of it. What does it taste like? What is the sensation of chewing and swallowing? Try to describe it to yourself in as much detail as possible and write down your observations below. Then write down what it was like for you to slow down and really pay attention. What did you notice?

_____

_____

_____

_____

_____

_____

_____

_____

This exercise is a classic savoring exercise, but it can be extended in many different ways. You can savor the feeling of the wind on your face as you take a walk, you can savor the sounds of the ocean or a bird singing. You can even savor the feel of a good belly laugh with friends. Savoring is a skill that can be built up over time, as you pay more attention to the lovely experiences in your day and what it's like to experience them in the present moment.

Try tracking your practice of the savoring skills for a few days, if you feel it'll be helpful for you.

What I savored: _____

What it was like: _____

_____

_____

_____

_____

What I savored: _____

What it was like: _____

_____

_____

_____

_____

What I savored: _____

What it was like: _____

_____

_____

_____

_____

What I savored: _____

What it was like: _____

_____

_____

_____

_____

Stop and Look Around

One of the quickest ways to practice savoring and stay grounded in the busy, information-rich world we live in is to immerse ourselves in nature. According to researchers (Ballew and Omoto 2018), sitting in the natural environment can increase our ability to savor and become completely absorbed. This can cultivate values related to being present, increasing awareness of small things, connecting with the environment and the planet, and taking a broader perspective than just what we focus on when we look at things through our ever-present thoughts.

EXERCISE: Stop and (Literally) Smell the Flowers

Find a natural space (woods, stream, park, beach, backyard with green in it) and sit and observe for twenty minutes. Do it alone, with no distractions—and no phone. (Yes, you read that correctly, no phone. We know it's tough, but trust us).

Utilize the same "sensory-perceptual sharpening" skills you used in the savoring exercise. Close your eyes and listen for a while. Notice the smells. Look close and see the small parts of the world you miss every day. Write down both what you noticed and what the experience was like.

_____

_____

_____

_____

_____

_____

_____

_____

_____

This exercise reminds us of something we know but often forget—we are not that important in the grand scheme of things. Spending time being present in nature allows us to recalibrate to our place in the world and connect to things that matter. And maybe experience a little awe.

Gratitude

When we talk about gratefulness and gratitude in everyday life, we're often talking about a trait (being a grateful person) or a mood (having feelings of gratitude). For our purposes here, it's more useful to think of gratitude as an active practice or set of behaviors. This can include the behavior of noticing benefits that are occurring in our lives, the behavior of acknowledging when things go well, the behavior of noticing what you have versus what you don't have, and the behavior of noticing all of the many helping hands you have in your life.

EXERCISE: Eternally Grateful

Want to increase your ability to notice when things go well? Here is an exercise for building that muscle.

In the table, right down twenty things about *your body* that you are grateful for right now. Be sure to write twenty things, even if you have a hard time thinking of them.

Something about my body	Why I'm grateful for it
1.	
2.	
3.	
4.	
5.	
6.	
7.	
8.	
9.	
10.	

Something about my body	Why I'm grateful for it
11.	
12.	
13.	
14.	
15.	
16.	
17.	
18.	
19.	
20.	

We tend to focus on the parts of our bodies that we don't like or wish were different. This exercise forces us to also notice the elements that we appreciate but might not consider.

While appreciating the well-working parts of our bodies might be particularly useful for some people, appreciating our bodies, specifically, isn't the point of this exercise. Rather, it's to demonstrate how to build the muscle of noticing things from multiple perspectives, including those we might not normally attend to. This same awareness building can be used for other areas, too, like music you appreciate, experiences you've had, choices you've made, lessons you've learned, and things that have worked out well when you thought they might not.

Gratitude for People in Your Life

Many of us aspire to be grateful to the people in our lives, but it is not always easy. Our default is often to notice the things that we don't appreciate about what people in our lives do, while we tend to not notice the things we might be grateful for. To counteract these tendencies, we can cultivate values and behaviors related to gratitude and thankfulness.

EXERCISE: Thank Your Lucky Star

When we want to cultivate our gratitude values, we can spend time thinking about all of the awesome fabulousness our loved ones have brought into our lives. Making room in our busy thoughts to really appreciate the cool things people have done for us—and then taking time to *express* gratitude to the people we're thankful for—is the purpose of this classic positive psychology exercise. This expression of gratitude, perhaps more than any single thing we can do in our relationships, builds connections, openness, and interdependence with those we love.

To start, think about someone who has benefited you in your life. Think about what your life would be like without them and think specifically about the things that they have done that have enhanced your experience in this life. Be as specific as possible.

Now write a heartfelt letter to the person thanking them. Again, being as specific as possible, write them a letter detailing the impact they have made on your life and the benefits they have brought to you. Express as clearly as you can your gratitude for all that they have done.

Once you have written the letter comes the hard part. For this exercise to positively impact your relationship, it is important to *read the letter to them*. We know, we know. This part of the exercise often makes people feel very uncomfortable and more than a little vulnerable. However, the benefits of the reading part of this exercise are clear: people who read the letter to the person they wrote about generally experience more lasting benefits than those who just write it. What a beautiful way to live your gratitude and connection values, while making room for discomfort and vulnerability. So lovely.

When you have written your letter and read it to the person you wrote it to, write down what you noticed for your future reference. What happened? How did the person respond to the letter? What did you notice for yourself as you wrote it, when you were reading it, and afterward?

_____

_____

_____

_____

_____

_____

_____

_____

_____

_____

Living Compassion Values

Another important positive value people often want to cultivate is that of compassion for others and for themselves. Compassion is talked about in many ways, but researchers (Strauss et al. 2016) have compiled a definition of compassion that can be particularly helpful in thinking about how to cultivate it. The elements of the definition include (1) recognizing suffering in oneself and others, (2) understanding the universality of suffering, (3) feeling sympathy, empathy, or concern for those who are suffering, (4) tolerating our own discomfort and distress in the presence of suffering, and (5) acting or being motivated to act to help those who are suffering.

As with the other topics in this chapter, it is important to remember that we are not talking necessarily about cultivating *feelings* of compassion. Instead, we want to think about what behaviors represent compassion, and how to best increase our awareness of them and cultivate our ability to engage in them. We also want to remember that everybody suffers from time to time. This will allow us to increase our ability to recognize people who are suffering, connect with them from a place of compassion and concern, and lean into them while making room for our own discomfort. It also helps us continue to understand that we're not alone in feeling what we feel—even if, in the hardest moments, it can seem that way.

When people struggle with difficult feelings in our presence, it is sometimes tempting to turn away from or turn down the volume of their suffering to protect ourselves. Ironically, showing compassion tends to lead to more vitality in our lives, even when it hurts our hearts.

Sending Good Vibes, the ACT Way

The following exercise develops our compassion muscle, while allowing us to cultivate the ability to send out "loving-kindness" and live our loving values, no matter what is happening.

Loving-kindness is a concept that is defined as the heartfelt wish for the well-being of oneself and all other beings (Salzberg 2004). It can be described as the softening of the heart that allows us to feel compassion for others and then wish them well. Traditional loving-kindness involves sending wishes of safety, peace, and happiness. Our "ACT take" on loving-kindness will include phrases designed to send out flexible awareness and meaningful values-based living.

There are many ways to cultivate loving-kindness, but the most common involves sitting in meditation and mentally repeating specific phrases designed to send loving-kindness to various people. In this exercise, we will first send loving-kindness (by repeating the specific phrases below) to a "benefactor." A benefactor is anybody who has been helpful to you, or anybody for whom it is very easy for you to feel love, without complication. This can be a loved one, a teacher, or even a pet.

Next, we will send loving-kindness to ourselves. This can be tricky for people sometimes. It can be easier to think of sending loving-kindness to the parts of you that are trying hard to live authentically.

Third, we will send loving-kindness to an acquaintance. This shouldn't be somebody you know well, but rather a neighbor or coworker whom you know, but not especially closely.

Finally, we will send loving-kindness to all beings.

On the days you're feeling ambitious, you can also send loving-kindness to somebody you struggle with—but as you're just starting out, or if you find yourself getting caught up in a story about that person or find it difficult to send them loving-kindness, save that for another day.

As the phrases are repeated, a sense of loving-kindness and goodwill can develop for all the people described, as well as people in general. It is quite amazing.

Sometimes, people do not find these phrases helpful for generating loving-kindness. In this case, it is also great to just think about the people, let the loving-kindness feelings develop as they will, and just send the sensations and the love out to all people instead of thinking of the actual phrases. We recommend you start with mentally repeating the phrases and see what happens.

EXERCISE: Sending Loving-Kindness

To start the exercise, find a comfortable place to sit and take a posture that is both relaxed and alert. With loving-kindness meditation, the priority is on self-care and comfort, so your posture for this meditation should be as loving toward yourself as possible, while still allowing you to stay focused on the task.

Set a timer for twenty minutes and close your eyes or soften your gaze on a spot on the floor in front of you.

Then, begin by sending loving-kindness to your benefactor. Remember, a benefactor can be a partner, child, friend, teacher, or even a pet. You don't need to know them personally, but they should be a being who has helped you and is easy to send love to. Slowly repeat the following phrases about ten times, while thinking of the benefactor, at a pace that feels comfortable to you:

May you be safe and know that you are safe.

May you be loved and know that you are loved.

May you have mindful awareness of your thoughts and see that they are thoughts.

May you live with intention.

Now, to send loving-kindness to yourself, your acquaintance, and the world, you will repeat the phrases about ten times toward each recipient at a pace that feels comfortable to you. Be sure to really think about the recipient each time, and really try to send the wish to them. Repeat as necessary until the timer goes off.

Once you're finished with your first practice, reflect What did you notice?

_____

_____

_____

_____

_____

_____

Living Forgiveness Values

There is an old saying that everybody in your life will eventually let you down (just as you will eventually let them down), and you only have control over how you respond to them when they do. While it is likely not true that *every single* person you meet or get to know in this life will let you down, or that you'll inevitably let down every single person you meet or get to know, we all know that human relationships are a wild jumble of missteps, reactivities, crossed priorities, and misunderstandings.

There are times when those missteps and crossed priorities lead to real hurt, or to a feeling that harm or injustice was done to us. We might feel lots of—perhaps justifiable—anger and hurt, and we might find ourselves getting lost in ruminative thoughts about it. Forgiveness isn't about forgetting about or glossing over harm or hurt feelings. It's about noticing these experiences and staying intentional rather than reactive.

Generally, the ACT approach to situations in which we've been or feel hurt involves all the skills we have targeted in the other chapters—coming into the present; noticing thoughts and feelings; deidentifying with self, defusion, acceptance, or willingness; and clarifying and moving toward personal values.

However, sometimes we don't have the skills to move toward our values (and behaviors) of forgiveness. Maybe this is because we never learned how to do so growing up, or maybe it is because we don't have practice with it, because when people hurt us in the past, we just cut them out of our lives. Whatever the reason, it is never too late to learn forgiveness skills—or to see what they might make possible for you as you seek to heal from harm.

EXERCISE: Gratitude in Harm?

Think about a time that somebody wronged you. Try to pick a situation that is not the most difficult thing that has happened to you, but a small- to medium-size hurt (we're just building muscles here).

In the space below, write about *the ways that experience has been good for your life* or allowed you to connect to or live your values. Rather than writing about the experience and what happened and how wrong it was, try to just write about what values-related lessons you have taken from the experience and any benefits you received from it. It is okay if that is not the perspective you have taken in the past—see if you can connect to ways the experience has strengthened your values of how you want to be or how you want to show up when somebody does something negative to you.

_____

_____

_____

_____

_____

_____

_____

_____

It is tempting to interpret the point of this exercise as to try to have more forgiving feelings or less pain and resentment. You might even have experienced either or both things. Changing feelings, however, is not the point of the exercise. The purpose of this exercise is to help you step back and see a difficult situation from multiple perspectives and think about it more broadly in terms of your values. This will not only give you more flexibility in responding to this situation or person, but will also allow you to build your forgiveness muscle to allow you to respond flexibly—rather than automatically—when people (inevitably) wrong you in the future.

Context Matters

Of course, when talking about forgiveness, context is particularly important. Cultivating forgiveness in the context of the common ups and downs of relationships—which is what we've been exploring here—is not the same as cultivating it in a context of abuse or mistreatment.

While it can be important to develop the ability to let go of small wrongs, it can also be important to leave a situation or relationship where you're experiencing real, lasting harm. If this applies to you, we encourage you to do what the situation demands, seeking help from friends or professionals as you need it.

Living Kindness and Generosity Values

Humans are social and interconnected beings. We need each other, and in some ways, we need to be needed by each other as well. When people list their personal values in ACT, "kind" and "generous" often make the list. But as common as these values are, finding ways to intentionally generate actions to go with them can be trickier, as we are often very involved with "me, myself, and mine" in our day-to-day existence.

So, if we are generally worried about ourselves, why do we so often wish to cultivate kindness and generosity? Humans have evolved in the context of social groups for the last fifty million years or so (Shulz, Opie, and Atkinson 2011), and it was crucially important for our survival to be thought of positively within those groups. Additionally, there are lots of studies demonstrating that behaving in kind and generous ways is related to higher levels of well-being and happiness (Curry et al. 2018). In fact, likely because of the evolutionary benefits, there are studies that show a bigger bump in well-being if we use our limited resources on others rather than on ourselves (Dunn et al. 2008).

Once again, however, utilizing generosity to improve mood is a tricky business. When we attempt to directly reduce our negative feelings and increase our positive feelings—even through something as lovely as generosity—we run the risk of running into the same problematic cycle addressed in the rest of this book. Instead, we can utilize the power of kindness and generosity by moving toward them as values, rather than pointedly seeking to move away from negative feelings or in search of positive ones.

EXERCISE: Random Acts of Kindness

Whether it's family, community, or just people in our world, humans have evolved to show kindness to one another. In this exercise, we will create concrete ways to live kindness and generosity values by setting an intention ahead of time.

Think about the people in your life and the people around you. Who is struggling? Who is trying to do something tough and could use some help and support? Who could use a friendly text or phone call? In the space below, create a menu of "kindness acts" you could take in your life right now.

Then (and here's the hard part), once a week for the next month, do five of these "kindness actions" in one day. For example, you could pick Saturdays as your day, and each Saturday, you would pick five acts and perform them all on that day.

Some people prefer to generate the list each week so that the kindness acts are the most relevant for what is happening, and that is fine too. The most important point to remember is that these should be extra—as much as possible, you should just live your life as you normally would, and just add in these days of five kind acts. Also, the goal is not to hold yourself to a standard of being generous all the time, every day. This is just a fun, once-weekly activity to organically kick your values of kindness and generosity into a higher gear.

Kindness Acts	

This exercise provides a structured way to think about and live your kindness values, which will let you bring more consistency to the cultivation of generosity. Remember, from an ACT perspective, the most important element of a practice like this is not the short-term improvement in mood you might gain, but rather the ability to consistently move toward values.

Living Love Values

Love is grand. It is a crucial part of human existence. But it is also difficult, painful, frustrating, and sometimes quite heartbreaking. Let's talk about how to develop skills for living our values related to closeness, connection, disclosure, vulnerability, and love.

Closeness

Research has long shown us that being disconnected from other people is not an optimal context for human beings (Jaremka and Sunami 2018). However, it wasn't until the COVID-19 pandemic brought forced "social distancing" to many parts of the world that these scientific findings hit home in a new way for many of us.

Living social connection and relationship values can be really hard. Even very supportive relationships tend to bring plenty of short-term stressors, and as we discussed in chapter 1, when our first response to emotions like stress is to avoid them at all costs, living social values can seem not worth the trouble. In addition, even when you want to have social connections, knowing how to cultivate close relationships and friendships can be difficult.

The Thing About Self-Disclosure

Have you ever noticed that the people you feel the closest to tend to be the people who know you best? It is the people who know us with all our quirks—the good, the bad, and the downright ugly—that we tend to feel the most connected to. And the opposite is also true, that the people we care about the most tend to be the people we know best, with all their good, bad, and ugly qualities. Partly, this is because the better we know somebody, the more we trust them with our less-than-Instagrammable moments. But researchers have been exploring the impact of self-disclosure on relationships, and they have discovered that the arrow may actually go in both directions.

In an early study on the topic, Aron and colleagues (1997) examined the effect of self-disclosure on relationship closeness through a procedure involving the asking and answering of increasingly personal questions. They found that even with strangers, asking and answering personal questions generated more closeness than small-talk questions that did not include self-disclosure.

EXERCISE: See and Be Seen

This exercise capitalizes on the research findings above, along with other research which has found that having genuine, self-disclosing discussions can increase the closeness of relationships.

Set aside time to talk with somebody who is important to you in your life and ask and answer each of the questions below. You can pick anybody you like to do the exercise with, but it should be somebody you have some level of trust with, and somebody you have an interest in connecting with or getting to know better.

Questions

1. What is your favorite thing about your life right now?

2. Who do you worry most about in your life?

3. If you could travel anywhere in the world, where would you go and why?

4. Who are you most grateful for? Why?

5. What was your favorite thing about your childhood? What do you most wish had been different?

6. What is your favorite guilty pleasure?

7. What is your biggest dream for the future?

8. If somebody looked in your purse/bag/wallet/room, what would they find?

9. If you could see the future, what is one thing you would want to know?

10. What are you most proud of?

11. What is your favorite thing about the person you are answering these questions with?

12. What do you have in common with the person you are answering these questions with? (Try to generate five true statements that start with "We both…")

The goal for this exercise isn't to get through the questions as quickly as possible or to know the most about one another. Instead, the benefit is in the process of sitting down together and sharing yourself and really learning about each other's inner lives. The ability to take risks and show ourselves in relationships is way more important to the value of closeness than knowing facts about each other.

Once you've finished the practice, come back to this workbook and write about the experience. What did you notice?

_____

_____

_____

_____

_____

_____

_____

_____

_____

. This exercise provides an opportunity to develop our relationships and closeness while practicing the skill of appropriate self-disclosure.

Summing It Up

As we've mentioned throughout this book, the main goal of ACT is to help change the responses to our thoughts and feelings to help us live a life that is more intentional and based on our values. Among those thoughts, feelings, and values are the many parts of life that are wonderful—joy, forgiveness, compassion, gratitude, connection, and kindness. Bringing awareness to the whole range of our human experience allows us to cultivate values related to these elements of life without excessive control or avoidance. Including the positive keeps us open to our whole realm of experience while staying focused on our most important values.

CHAPTER 8

Bringing It All Together

Living Flexibly

Let's sum this all up. In chapter 1, we learned about the relationship between avoidance and control, and the ACT alternative to excessively trying to control thoughts and feelings: psychological flexibility. Psychological flexibility involves six processes, which we shared with you across chapters 2 to 7. We then added some skills from the positive psychology tradition that we think go really well with values and committed action, and can help you enhance your practice of building a meaningful life. Throughout this book, we have tried to not just introduce you to ideas intellectually—though there's been plenty of that—but also introduce you to ideas experientially. So, let's bring this together a pair of exercises that capture psychological flexibility as a whole. The first is an embodied metaphor of psychological flexibility introduced by ACT cofounder Steve Hayes (2019).

EXERCISE: Two Postures

Get ready to do something a little different. Like some of the exercises throughout this book, it's going to involve getting closer to something that might be a bit painful. Pick something you struggle with that you're willing to spend a little time on. It doesn't have to be the hardest thing you experience. But it helps if it's something meaningful that is the source of some internal suffering, like the examples you've worked with throughout the book.

Let's start by briefly coming into the present moment.

First, tune into the sounds in your environment. Notice the variety of sounds across the landscape of your hearing for the next thirty seconds, then read the next paragraph.

Next, tune into the sensations where your body makes contact with the chair or surface on which you're sitting, and notice the variety of sensations there. Let your attention linger there for the next thirty seconds or so before reading on.

Now tune in to your breath, watching the rising and falling in your body, just observing the sensations as you breathe in and breathe out. And let your attention linger there for about half a minute.

When you're ready, call to mind a place in your life where you struggle in some way. It doesn't have to be the hardest place, just something that seems meaningful. When you've got it, call up some representation of it in your imagination—an image, a thought, or a memory—and hold it there for the next few moments.

Now, adopt a posture with your body that captures how you are when you're responding at your worst with that struggle. In other words, let your body represent what you're like when you're responding at your worst. And as you do that, just notice what it's like.

After thirty seconds, feel free to return to neutral.

Next, adopt a posture that captures how you are when you're responding at your best with that struggle. The struggle is still there, but you are responding at your best.

And just notice what *that* is like.

Now, allow your posture to go back to neutral and let the image go. Tune back into this moment by noticing the sounds in your environment and the sensations where your body meets the chair before reading on.

Finally, before we debrief, offer yourself a small gesture of gratitude for being willing to get close to pain for a moment.

What did you notice?

_____

_____

_____

_____

_____

_____

_____

Most people pick two postures. At their worst, they are bending over in some way, often covering their faces, and making themselves smaller. Think of a child bending over in tears. At their best, they are looking up with arms spread wide, in a gesture that suggests openness and receptiveness.

Notice how the first one is closed, narrow, and small. The second one is open, broad, and bigger. If you didn't adopt these exact postures, that's okay. People often come up with different ones. But let's stay with looking at these two examples here for a moment.

Notice that we didn't invite you to imagine postures that represented the difference between how you are or how you feel when the problem is present or absent. We invited you to imagine two different responses to the problem. Sometimes we have no choice about whether some difficulty is present, whether it's inside of us, like shame, anxiety, or self-critical thinking, or in our lives, like a conflict with someone we love or a difficult situation at work. But we can choose how we *respond*. We can respond in a way that helps us, or we can respond in a way that makes things more difficult. Responding in a way that works for our lives is what psychological flexibility is all about.

EXERCISE: Worst Responses, Best Responses

Let's make this concrete by focusing on behavior. Map out what you typically do when you are responding at your worst or at your best. What does that look like *in your actions?* If you need to see an example, Matt has one, after the exercise, related to a problem in his life: his tendency to feel blue when things slow down at the end of the workweek and his mind has time to wander.

Problem: _____

	Responding at my worst	**Responding at my best**
What is my mind focused on?		
What am I doing (i.e., what actions am I taking)?		
What words would describe my behavior?		

Problem: Waking up feeling blue on a Saturday morning

	Responding at my worst	**Responding at my best**
What is my mind focused on?	I focus on my fatigue and my worries about what the rest of the day will be like.	I focus on mapping out a day that is about rest and self-care.
What am I doing?	I move distractedly between one halfhearted task and another—emptying the dishwasher, making coffee, picking up around the house, looking at my phone.	I start with a to do list and organize my day around not just household tasks, but also being creative and having fun—writing music, going out for coffee with my wife, getting outdoors for a bit. As I do those things, I do my best to be present to what I'm doing, even if my mood continues to get my attention.
What words would describe my behavior?	Going through the motions	Active, engaged, purposeful

In both the left and right columns, the blue mood is still there, though you can probably guess that when he's responding in the way described on the right, the blue mood is more likely to dissipate throughout the day. And even if it lingers—because it sometimes does—there are other experiences that go along with it: moments of pleasure and delight, moments of connection with others, and feelings of accomplishment.

Psychological flexibility doesn't assume that uncomfortable thoughts and feelings won't be present. In fact, it predicts that they will be present, no matter what we are doing. The question becomes, what do we do when they show up? What is directing our lives? Are we simply fighting these thoughts and feelings, or following where they lead? Or are we doing something that captures a bigger picture—where we truly want to be?

Some people remember to respond flexibly by keeping these postures in mind. Others use terms like "open, aware, active," a nifty shorthand for the lengthy—and admittedly cumbersome—ACT flexibility processes: acceptance, defusion, present moment awareness, self-as-context, values, and committed action. Here are some other ways to bring flexibility into your life by drawing on all of these processes without having to pause and think, "Wait, do I start with values? Or do I start with defusion? What's the difference between present moment awareness and flexible perspective taking?"

The ACT Matrix

In the early days of ACT—or, really, the early public days of ACT, when therapists from outside a few small psychological laboratories were experimenting with it—clinicians began to develop their own innovations within the ACT model. Kevin Polk, along with colleagues Jerold Hambright and Mark Webster, began imagining a visual representation of ACT they could use to make it easy for anyone to understand. And thus, the ACT Matrix, was born.

The ACT Matrix is a four-quadrant grid that helps people understand how avoidance and control might take them away from what's meaningful to them. It has since been transported and adapted all around the world for widely different problems (Polk et al. 2016), even showing up in ACT research (Arch et al. 2019). In some versions, it's completely turned upside down (literally, e.g., Hayes 2019), yet it still captures the heart of what the matrix has to offer: a visual overview of how your behavior works. So, the following is just one way to do the ACT Matrix, and you may encounter it looking very different in other ACT books. This one starts with Polk's model, but has influences from the adaptation by Joanna Arch and her team at University of Colorado, and ACT trainer Lou Lasprugato, who uses it regularly.

EXERCISE: ACT Matrix

You can either do this exercise in reference to your life as a whole, or if that's a bit complicated, pick a specific area of your life such as your career, your relationship with a friend, or the way you look after your health.

Start by thinking of this as a perspective-taking exercise. You are stepping back and looking at patterns of your behavior from a bird's-eye view. You could think of the "me noticing" bubble as the observer's perspective.

Begin the exercise with the box on bottom right and go counterclockwise, filling out the relevant details. You'll begin with your values. Who and what is important to you? How do you want to be in your actions? Then you'll move to inner struggles, away moves, and finally to toward moves. Notice that the stuff on the bottom is stuff that occurs inside of you—mental and emotional things like your values and your thoughts and feelings. The stuff on the top consists of actions that could be observable to anyone— your actions, what you do with your hands, feet, and voice. If you would like to see an example of a matrix that's already been completed, take a look at Camille's matrix a couple pages later.

AWAY *from pain*   **Outside**   **TOWARD** *meaning and purpose*

Away moves

*What do you do to **get away** from inner struggles? And what do you do when inner struggles guide your actions?*

Toward moves

*What have you done or could you do to **move toward** (e.g., cct on) your values?*

ME NOTICING

Inner struggles

What thoughts and feelings get in the way of moving toward your values (e.g., anxiety, sadness, physical pain, shame, "I'll never be good enough," "I can't trust anyone")?

Values

What's important to you? What qualities do you want to bring to your actions (e.g., prioritizing family, making a difference in the world, being compassionate, building meaningful relationships)?

Inside

Away moves. "Away moves" are actions that we take to diminish the power of or have more control over our inner struggles—in other words, they take us away from pain. Notice the relationship between the bottom left and the top left: the actions on the top left often diminish the intensity of the experiences on the bottom left in the short term, but can lead to greater intensity and persistence in the long term. It's a vicious cycle: it's like scratching a mosquito bite or licking your lips when they are chapped.

Toward moves. "Toward moves" are values-based behaviors—i.e., moving toward your values in your actions. The matrix can be a great place to see whether or not you are putting energy into your life in meaningful ways, and where you could be doing more or doing something differently. In any given moment, about any behavior, you can ask yourself, "Is this an away move? Is it a toward move?"

Toward values, away from pain. The words "toward" and "away" can confuse people into thinking that the matrix asks you to label behavior as toward and away from values or toward and away from pain. Some later matrix adaptations indeed do this. However, we have stuck to the original model, which is *toward values* and *away from pain*.

Workability: Notice that the same behavior can be an away move or a toward move depending on the context. No action is in and of itself a toward move or an away move. That's where workability comes in. For most of us, leaving a job that makes us miserable is a toward move, but it's also an away move.

For some of us, taking a nap is a delightful treat. For others, it's an escape from difficult feelings. And for still others, it can be either, depending on the day.

There is no right way to act. Avoid making a false binary between toward moves and away moves, in which toward moves are good and away moves are bad. That's not what this perspective is about. It's about developing an understanding of your behavior and then using that understanding to have more freedom to choose and act.

Camille's Example

Way back in chapter 1, we introduced you to Camille. We gave you a brief thumbnail of her behavior to describe how avoidance and control were making her life more difficult. Here's what we wrote:

> *Camille feels anxious in groups, especially at work. She rarely goes out with her colleagues and doesn't speak up in meetings. She doesn't want people to see her face flushing when she talks, and she doesn't like the feeling of her heart racing. As a result, she feels disconnected from her colleagues, who don't really know her—or her great ideas—very well. And the anxiety persists.*

Let's flesh this out into a matrix about her whole life, taking into account some additional details about her life that we haven't shared yet.

AWAY *from pain*   **Outside**   **TOWARD** *meaning and purpose*

Toward moves

What have you done or could you do to **move toward** *(e.g., act on) your values?*

Exercise

Spending time with my nieces and family

Perhaps going back to school to further my career?

Being a more integral part of work projects

Saying yes to invitations

ME NOTICING

Values

What's important to you? What qualities do you want to bring to your actions (e.g., prioritizing family, making a difference in the world, being compassionate, building meaningful relationships)?

Being a good auntie to my nieces

Being loyal to my family

Having a meaningful career

Finding a partner and building a family someday

Volunteering at church

Being kind to other people

Crafting

Away moves

What do you do to **get away** *from inner struggles? And what do you do when inner struggles guide your actions?*

Not speaking up at work

Not taking invitations to go out with colleagues

Avoiding pursuing a relationship

Isolating myself when I get really sad or anxious

Exercise

Prayer

Inner struggles

What thoughts and feelings get in the way of moving toward your values (e.g., anxiety, sadness, physical pain, shame, "I'll never be good enough," "I can't trust anyone")?

Anxiety about not doing it right at work, at church, and with family

Racing heart

Comparing myself to other people

"They will see my hands shaking if I speak up at work."

"They won't like me if they get to know me better."

"I can't date until I lose some weight."

Always wondering if there's something wrong with me

Inside

Let's notice a few preliminary things about Camille's matrix. First of all, it's a moment in time. She might do it again tomorrow and come up with a few different words. Also, she is taking a bird's-eye view of her whole life. She could go deeper by doing a narrower matrix on her relationship with family, her work life, her dating life, or even a difficult conversation with a friend that she is anticipating. I (Matt) get the most out of using the matrix around specific situations. What are my values in this moment? How do I want to show up? And how might I work against those values if I'm not paying attention?

As we go deeper, we can notice, as we have been noticing throughout the whole book, that stuff on the top left probably works in the short term to make the stuff on the bottom left go away. But it probably doesn't do so in the long term. And though we haven't written them down, you can probably imagine some costs for the actions on the top left.

Next, let's notice that some of the stuff on the top left is the same as the stuff on the top right (exercise, prayer, therapy). Her job might be to notice when these behaviors are more directed toward escaping thoughts and feelings and less directed toward building the life she wants. Therapy, for example, can be about simply spinning your wheels when there's no action attached to it.

Finally, the matrix doesn't tell her what to do. Remember that circle in the middle? It's just a way to notice, and in that noticing, perhaps her perspective expands, and her possibilities for acting become more varied, fearless, and values driven. And making those choices might be a little bit easier with the help of the skills in this book, a similar workbook, a good therapist, or a good friend.

A Benediction

As we wrap up *The ACT Skills Workbook*, we would like to leave you with a benediction. A benediction, whether in a religious or nonreligious setting, is an expression of good wishes. You may be familiar with the traditional Irish benediction, a version of which goes, "May the road rise to meet you. May the wind be always at your back. May the sun shine warm upon your face. And rains fall soft upon your fields" (Wilson 2023). Here's ours for you, which is centered around the themes of this book:

May you live a life of meaning and purpose, whatever burdens or joys you may be carrying in this moment.

May you show up to your internal pain with just enough openness to make greater things possible in your life.

May you learn to use your most amazing tool—your mind—without letting it pull you away into believing everything it says.

May you carry a sense of you that is bigger than whatever you feel in the moment, bigger than the stories that you and others tell about you, and bigger than any event that has happened in your life.

May you notice happiness, gratitude, awe, compassion, and any other quality that might enhance and enrichen your life.

May you know the present moment, and in the present moment, may you find beauty.

Matt and Jen, 2024

Evidence-Based ACT
Self-Help Books

Here are some evidence-based ACT self-help books that have been researched in randomized controlled trials as a standalone intervention.

Get Out of Your Mind and Into Your Life by Steven C. Hayes and Spencer Smith

The Mindfulness and Acceptance Workbook for Anxiety by John P. Forsyth and Georg H. Eifert

The Mindfulness and Acceptance Workbook for Social Anxiety and Shyness by Jan E. Fleming and Nancy L. Kocovski

The Mindful Way Through Anxiety by Susan M. Orsillo and Lizabeth Roemer

Acknowledgments

We'd like to thank all of people we have served in our clinical work over the past twenty-five years, each of whom have allowed us to be with them in their struggles and growth. We are grateful to our mentors, colleagues, friends, and everyone else we have learned from in the ACT and greater contextual behavioral science communities, including Steve Hayes, Robyn Walser, Kelly Wilson, Lisa Coyne, Emily Sandoz, Melissa Londoño Connally, R. Sonia Singh, John Forsyth, Russ Harris, Spencer Smith, Troy Dufrene, Lou Lasprugato, Jennifer Payne, Louise McHugh, Rikki Kjelgaard, Louise Hayes, Liz Gifford, Martin Brock, Joanne Dahl, and JT Blackledge. We are also grateful to the team at New Harbinger, especially Elizabeth Hollis Hansen, Vicraj Gill, M. C. Calvi, and Catharine Meyers. Thanks also to Jim Harper and Jan Dean for commenting on the flexible perspective taking chapter. An enormous thank you goes to Praxis Continuing Education and Training for giving us a platform to train other therapists and allowing us to adapt content from Matt's *ACT Basics* online training for this book. Finally, we'd like to thank our families: Glenn, Hope, and Jack, Sandie, Sue, Larry, Julie, Gail, Wayne, Ben, Kendra, Mari, Neil, Lori, Taylor, Shane, Jesse, Matt, Kierra, Lily, Toni Jaudon, Giorgia, Finley, and the entire extended Boonedoggle.

References

Acarturk, C., E. Uygun, Z. Ilkkursun, K. Carswell, F. Tedeschi, M. Batu, et al. 2022. "Effectiveness of a WHO Self-Help Psychological Intervention for Preventing Mental Disorders Among Syrian Refugees in Turkey: A Randomized Controlled Trial." *World Psychiatry* 21: 88–95.

Arch, J. J., J. L. Mitchell, S. R. Genung, R. Fisher, D. J. Andorsky, and A. L. Stanton. 2019. "A Randomized Controlled Trial of a Group Acceptance-Based Intervention for Cancer Survivors Experiencing Anxiety at Re-Entry ('Valued Living'): Study Protocol." *BMC Cancer* 19: 1–11.

Aron, A., E. Melinat, E. N. Aron, R. D. Vallone, and R. J. Bator. 1997. "The Experimental Generation of Interpersonal Closeness: A Procedure and Some Preliminary Findings." *Personality and Social Psychology Bulletin* 23: 363–377.

Association for Contextual Behavioral Science (ACBS). n.d. "ACT Studies in Low and Middle Income Countries." https://contextualscience.org/act_studies_in_low_and_middle_income_countries.

Ballew, M. T., and A. M. Omoto. 2018. "Absorption: How Nature Experiences Promote Awe and Other Positive Emotions." *Ecopsychology* 10: 26–35.

Boone, M. S. 2013. "Acceptance and Commitment Therapy (ACT): Theory and Individual Treatment." In *Acceptance and Mindfulness for Counseling College Students: Theory and Practical Applications for Intervention, Prevention, and Outreach*, edited by J. Pistorello. Oakland, CA: New Harbinger Publications.

Chase, J. A., R. Houmanfar, S. C. Hayes, T. A. Ward, J. Plumb Vilardaga, and V. Follette. 2013. "Values Are Not Just Goals: Online ACT-Based Values Training Adds to Goal Setting in Improving Undergraduate College Student Performance." *Journal of Contextual Behavioral Science* 2: 79–84.

Curry, O. S., L. A. Rowland, C. J. Van Lissa, S. Zlotowitz, J. McAlaney, and H. Whitehouse. 2018. "Happy to Help? A Systematic Review and Meta-Analysis of the Effects of Performing Acts of Kindness on the Well-Being of the Actor." *Journal of Experimental Social Psychology* 76: 320–329.

Dahl, J. 2015. "Valuing in ACT." *Current Opinion in Psychology* 2: 43–46.

Dunn, E., L. B. Aknin, and M. I. Norton. 2008. "Spending Money on Others Promotes Happiness." *Science* 319: 1687–1688.

Gloster, A. T., N. Walder, M. E. Levin, M. P. Twohig, and M. Karekla. 2020. "The Empirical Status of Acceptance and Commitment Therapy: A Review of Meta-Analyses." *Journal of Contextual Behavioral Science* 18: 181–192.

Harris, R. 2008. *The Happiness Trap: How to Stop Struggling and Start Living.* Boston: Trumpeter Books.

Hayes, S. C. 2019. *A Liberated Mind: How to Pivot Toward What Matters.* New York: Avery.

Hayes, S. C., K. D. Strosahl, and K. G. Wilson. 1999. *Acceptance and Commitment Therapy: An Experiential Approach to Behavior Change.* New York: Guilford Press.

Jansen, J. E., J. Gleeson, S. Bendall, S. Rice, and M. Alvarez-Jimenez. 2020. "Acceptance- and Mindfulness-Based Interventions for Persons with Psychosis: A Systematic Review and Meta-Analysis." *Schizophrenia Research* 215: 25–37.

Jaremka, L. M., and N. Sunami. 2018. "Threats to Belonging Threaten Health: Policy Implications for Improving Physical Well-Being." *Policy Insights from the Behavioral and Brain Sciences* 5: 90–97.

Kabat-Zinn, J. 1994. *Wherever You Go, There You Are: Mindfulness Meditation in Everyday Life.* New York: Hyperion.

King, L. A. 2001. "The Health Benefits of Writing About Life Goals." *Personality and Social Psychology Bulletin* 27: 798–807.

Masuda, A., S. C. Hayes, C. F. Sackett, and M. P. Twohig. 2004. "Cognitive Defusion and Self-Relevant Negative Thoughts: Examining the Impact of a Ninety Year Old Technique." *Behaviour Research and Therapy* 42: 477–485.

Mauss, I. B., N. S. Savino, C. L. Anderson, M. Weisbuch, M. Tamir, and M. L. Laudenslager. 2012. "The Pursuit of Happiness Can Be Lonely." *Emotion* 12: 908–912.

Mauss, I. B., M. Tamir, C. L. Anderson, and N. S. Savino. 2011. "Can Seeking Happiness Make People Unhappy? Paradoxical Effects of Valuing Happiness." *Emotion* 11: 807–815.

McGrath, J. J., A. Al-Hamzawi, J. Alonso, Y. Altwaijri, L. H. Andrade, E. J. Bromet, et al. 2023. "Age of Onset and Cumulative Risk of Mental Disorders: A Cross-National Analysis of Population Surveys from 29 Countries." *The Lancet Psychiatry* 10: 668–681.

Musanje, K., C. S. Camlin, M. R. Kamya, W. Vanderplasschen, D. L. Sinclair, M. Getahun, et al. 2023. "Culturally Adapting a Mindfulness and Acceptance-Based Intervention to Support the Mental Health of Adolescents on Antiretroviral Therapy in Uganda." *PLOS Global Public Health* 3: e0001605.

Muto, T., S. C. Hayes, and T. Jeffcoat. 2011. "The Effectiveness of Acceptance and Commitment Therapy Bibliotherapy for Enhancing the Psychological Health of Japanese College Students Living Abroad." *Behavior Therapy* 42: 323–335.

Páez-Blarrina, M., C. Luciano, O. Gutiérrez-Martínez, S. Valdivia, J. Ortega, and M. Rodríguez-Valverde. 2008. "The Role of Values with Personal Examples in Altering the Functions of Pain: Comparison Between Acceptance-Based and Cognitive-Control-Based Protocols." *Behaviour Research and Therapy* 46: 84–97.

Polk, K. L., B. Schoendorff, M. Webster, and F. O. Olaz. 2016. *The Essential Guide to the ACT Matrix: A Step-by-Step Approach to Using the ACT Matrix Model in Clinical Practice.* Oakland, CA: New Harbinger Publications.

Ritzert, T. R., J. P. Forsyth, S. C. Sheppard, J. F. Boswell, C. R. Berghoff, and G. H. Eifert. 2016. "Evaluating the Effectiveness of ACT for Anxiety Disorders in a Self-Help Context: Outcomes from a Randomized Wait-List Controlled Trial." *Behavior Therapy* 47: 444–459.

Salzberg, S. 2004. *Lovingkindness: The Revolutionary Art of Happiness.* Berkeley, CA: Shambhala Publications.

Seligman, M. E. 2011. *Flourish: A Visionary New Understanding of Happiness and Well-Being.* New York: Free Press.

Shultz, S., C. Opie, and Q. D. Atkinson. 2011. "Stepwise Evolution of Stable Sociality in Primates." *Nature* 479: 219–222.

Strauss, C., B. L. Taylor, J. Gu, W. Kuyken, R. Baer, F. Jones, and K. Cavanagh. 2016. "What Is Compassion and How Can We Measure It? A Review of Definitions and Measures." *Clinical Psychology Review* 47: 15–27.

Wegner, D. M. 1994. "Ironic Processes of Mental Control." *Psychological Review* 101: 34–52.

Wenzlaff, R. M., and D. M. Wegner. 2000. "Thought Suppression." *Annual Review of Psychology* 51: 59–91.

Wilson, J. 2023. "'May the Road Rise Up to Meet You'—The Story Behind the Traditional Irish Blessing." Irish Central. https://www.irishcentral.com/culture/may-the-road-rise-meet-you-irish-blessing-meaning.

World Health Organization. 2022. *Mental Health and COVID-19: Early Evidence of the Pandemic's Impact.* Scientific Brief: 2 March 2022. https://www.who.int/publications-detail-redirect/WHO-2019-nCoV-Sci_Brief-Mental_health-2022.1.

Matthew S. Boone, LCSW, is a social worker, psychotherapist, and educator who specializes in translating mental health concepts for the general public. Boone is a nationally recognized, peer-reviewed trainer in acceptance and commitment therapy (ACT), coauthor of *Stop Avoiding Stuff*, and editor of *Mindfulness and Acceptance in Social Work*. He is associate director of student mental health services at the University of Arkansas for Medical Sciences, where he is an instructor in psychiatry. He regularly gives ACT workshops around the country.

Jennifer Gregg, PhD, is a psychologist, author, professor, and trainer. She is a professor at San Jose State University, and has spent twenty years treating cancer patients and their families. Gregg has been studying, delivering, and evaluating ACT since 1995, and she has published dozens of research papers, book chapters, and articles on ACT. She is coauthor of *Stop Avoiding Stuff* and *The Diabetes Workbook*.

Foreword writer **Steven C. Hayes, PhD,** is Nevada Foundation Professor in the department of psychology at the University of Nevada, Reno; and author of nearly fifty books, including *Get Out of Your Mind and Into Your Life*. He has shown in his research how language and thought lead to human suffering, and is originator and codeveloper of ACT.

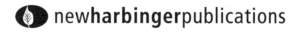

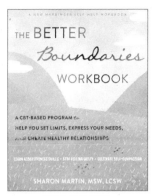
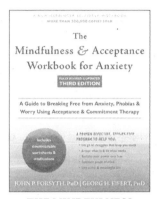
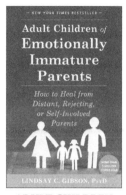
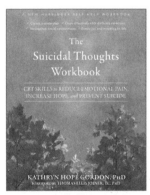
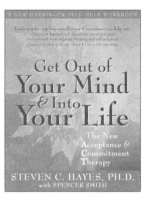
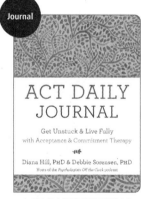

Did you know there are **free tools** you can download for this book?

Free tools are things like **worksheets**, **guided meditation exercises**, and **more** that will help you get the most out of your book.

You can download free tools for this book— whether you bought or borrowed it, in any format, from any source—from the New Harbinger website. All you need is a NewHarbinger.com account. Just use the URL provided in this book to view the free tools that are available for it. Then, click on the "download" button for the free tool you want, and follow the prompts that appear to log in to your NewHarbinger.com account and download the material.

You can also save the free tools for this book to your **Free Tools Library** so you can access them again anytime, just by logging in to your account! Just look for this button on the book's free tools page.

+ Save this to my free tools library

If you need help accessing or downloading free tools, visit **newharbinger.com/faq** or contact us at **customerservice@newharbinger.com**.